DATE DUE

Early-Stage Alzheimer's Care

Diane Weddington received her B.A. from Duke University, an M.A. from the University of Missouri–Columbia School of Journalism, and a Master of Divinity (M.Div.) from Duke Divinity School. She is a member of the American Academy of Religion, the Society of Professional Journalists, Women in Communications, and Religion Newswriters. She has been a Poynter Institute Fellow in Ethics and an American Press Institute Fellow in Aging.

Early-Stage Alzheimer's Care

A Guide for Community-Based Programs

Diane Weddington, MA, MDiv

Springer Publishing Company

Springer Publishing Company, Inc.
536 Broadway
New York, NY 10012

Cover design by Tom Yabut
Production Editor: Joyce Noulas

94 95 96 97 98 / 5 4 3 2 1

Library of Congress Cataloging-in-Publication Data

Weddington, Diane.
    Early-stage Alzheimer's care: a guide for community-based pro-
grams / Diane Weddington.
        p.   cm.
    Includes bibliographical references and index.
    ISBN 0-8261-8640-8
    1. Alzheimer's disease—Patients—Services for—Planning.
    2. Alzheimer's disease—Patients—Care.   3. Alzheimer's dis-
ease—Patients—Services for—United States.   I. Title.
    RC523.W43   1994
    362.1'96831—dc20   94-30812
                                                              CIP

Printed in the United States of America

Contents

Preface

This book has three purposes. The first is to provide information for people who plan to start early intervention programs for Alzheimer's disease patients. There is an urgent need for this information. The problem behaviors associated with the early stage can be reduced if intervention is prompt.

It is only in the past 5 years that early intervention programs have been established. Most of the material written about these programs is either unpublished or circulated to a limited audience. This book assimilates these materials, compares methods, and offers options. It summarizes the experiences of many professionals so that readers can learn what methods have worked and can get on with designing and setting up their own programs.

The second purpose of this volume is to provide a new resource for the families and friends of patients. Their concerns have a major impact on any program and it would have been impossible to write a book that did not include those concerns. Other books for caregivers are both abundant and adequate and people should turn to them for support during the *duration* of the disease. However, this book is useful in dealing with the first shock and the decision to seek out an *early* intervention program.

This volume's third purpose is to present the patient as a person who still has abilities, emotions, and plans, and who deserves autonomy, respect, and compassion. To that end, this book discusses myths about Alzheimer's disease, behaviors that can be expected, and strategies to deal with them.

Early-Stage Alzheimer's Care: A Guide for Community-Based Programs is organized according to the way issues should arise. Chapter 1 explains how Alzheimer's disease is diagnosed. It provides basic information about the difficulty of early-stage diagnosis.

Chapters 2 and 3 cover the practical aspects of starting a program, including choosing a site, raising funds, and hiring a staff.

Chapter 4 explains family issues that should be resolved or addressed before a patient enrolls in a program. Chapter 5 explains how to screen candidates.

Chapters 6 and 7 are devoted to practical aspects of conducting a program. Chapter 6 details the kinds of problem behaviors that are typical and ways to cope with them. Chapter 7 compares different kinds of programs and describes a range of activities that can be employed.

Chapter 8 briefly explains the issues that arise for everyone when a program ends.

The Appendix contains a limited number of resources. There is a list of early intervention programs. Also included are two forms which program directors can use to evaluate patients: the Mini-Mental State Exam, and a tool devised by the Honolulu, HI early stage group. Last, the appendix contains a sample of a durable power of attorney for health care. This form may help families or directors think about the issues that will arise when the program ends.

My work on this volume began as a plan to write a manual for The DRC Club of Walnut Creek, California. I took part in that program and learned by personal interaction some of the facts and fantasies about early-stage intervention. The DRC Club Board envisioned a manual that limited itself to a description of that program.

I realized the six women whom I observed represented only a small part of the affected population; their experiences and responses were qualified by their unique cultural, social, and geographical concerns. I also knew several men with early-stage dementia and they had different concerns, so I assumed that a program for men would be different, as would a program with both sexes. The structure and goals of the DRC Club reflected the singular knowledge and preferences of the program director. I knew that other equally valid approaches existed and that The DRC Club was not the first or only early intervention program.

I expanded the proposal, sent it to numerous publishers, and received an overwhelming response. I chose a publisher and set about writing a volume that would synthesize what I knew from personal experience and what I learned from printed materials. I was greatly aided in the latter process by members of a committee of the Greater San Francisco Bay Area Alzheimer's Association who surveyed early intervention programs in 1993 and helped me update what I knew from a 1991 national survey.

This book encompasses an array of models, theories, experiences, and issues. It does not attempt to promote any single program, nor would it be useful if it did. Ultimately each program will reflect the choices of its own team. What this book does is enlarge the choices.

Acknowledgments

I thank the board of the Diablo Respite Center in Walnut Creek, CA for allowing me to take part in their first early care program, the DRC Club. I am grateful to six patients who acted with bravery and dignity in the face of their diagnosis for sharing with me their struggle with the disease. I particularly thank Marilyn Trabert, Director of the DRC Club, who first suggested the need for this book.

I am especially grateful for the professional insights and personal support of Connee Pence, who has directed programs for Alzheimer's patients for more than a decade. I have been guided by Connee's belief that every person affected by dementia is also a person who deserves respect.

I am also grateful for the advice of the professionals in the San Francisco Bay Area whose knowledge and experience of the disease far exceeds mine. I particularly thank Bonnie Eisenberg, Julie Peck, Linda Fodrini-Johnson, and Joan Larsen, who are all passionately committed to the welfare of the elderly and the education of the public.

I learned valuable information from the unpublished work of David Wylie of the Greater San Francisco Bay Area Alzheimer's

Association and Robyn Yale, a licensed clinical social worker who has worked extensively with early stage patients.

I thank Dr. Jean LaTorre, a research psychologist for the Clorox Corporation, for reading parts of the manuscript.

I owe major thanks to Craig Von Bargen, Jeanie Wakeland, and their son David Von Bargen for giving me full access to their home and computer so I could prepare this manuscript.

I am also grateful for the support of Springer Publishing. I am honored that Dr. Ursula Springer believed that this book is important and that she trusted me to write it. I am particularly grateful for the assistance of my editor, Bill Tucker.

Most of all I thank Dr. C. E. Christian, a friend who believed more than I ever did that this book would actually be published. This book is dedicated to her with my deepest respect and gratitude.

D. W.

Introduction: Diagnosis of Early Alzheimer's Disease

1

Julia Sugarbaker, a character in the television comedy series "Designing Women," is the owner of a home interior design business. Typically she is portrayed as a level-headed feminist. In one episode she began to behave in ways that puzzled her partners. She would disappear for hours then lie about where she had been, she ordered tasteless flamboyant clothing she would not normally wear, and she began to neglect daily business matters. In short, her behavior changed abruptly and radically.

None of her partners knew she was moonlighting as a cabaret singer. Her absences were for practice sessions, the clothing was a stage costume, and she was distracted because she was trying to hide her private life from her partners. Not knowing any of this, her sister Suzanne came up with a different solution. Julia obviously had a disease that was affecting her mind. Suzanne Sugarbaker called it "Oldtimer's disease."

The scene is funny, but provides an ideal starting point for a discussion of Alzheimer's disease since it exemplifies common misconceptions about the disease.

Suzanne was certain she understood Julia's problem. She believed her sister had suddenly lost her mind. However, Alzheimer's disease takes a long time to do its damage. The patient's unusual behavior goes on for a long time and inevitably worsens.

Julia's strange behavior had a reasonable explanation. She did not have a permanent change in personality. Once her secret was discovered her partners no longer worried about her taste in clothing or her inattention to the business because they knew her behavior was temporary. Julia could still manage business affairs but was temporarily distracted.

By contrast, a real Alzheimer's disease patient would find it increasingly impossible to perform routine tasks. As Alzheimer's disease worsens, reason and logic disappear permanently.

Finally, Suzanne was only partly correct in calling the problem "Oldtimers' disease." Alzheimer's disease is primarily a disease of the aged, but can begin in mid-life. Interestingly, Suzanne was willing to use the label—an incomplete description of those affected by the disease—for her middle-aged sister.

As this scenario illustrates, any discussion of early Alzheimer's disease must be qualified.

On the one hand, health-care professionals agree upon a general list of behaviors and symptoms characteristic of the disease. On the other, behaviors and symptoms vary with each individual; there is no typical early stage patient.

Nor can early Alzheimer's disease be identified by duration. Whereas a heart attack is a climactic episode, Alzheimer's disease has an insidious progression. The course of the disease varies from a few months to 25 years.

Even making a diagnosis is difficult. The cause of the disease is unknown and it cannot be cured. The disease is readily confused with depression, delirium, other dementia, and even normal aging. These conditions can be ruled out by extensive neurological and mental testing, but a definite diagnosis can only be confirmed by a brain biopsy after death.

Diagnostic criteria have been set in light of these qualifications.

This chapter will examine those criteria and explain how an early stage patient is identified.

THE FIRST SIGNS

Alzheimer's disease was first diagnosed and described in 1907 by the German physician Alois Alzheimer. It is an irreversible, progressive, degenerative brain disease. A form of dementia, it impairs memory, thinking, and behavior. There is no cure and it is always fatal.

Like Suzanne Sugarbaker, most people know very little about Alzheimer's disease. Most people harbor fears about getting the disease, usually disguised in jokes about memory loss. Losing the keys or forgetting to send someone a birthday card provokes jokes about having Alzheimer's disease.

Short-term memory loss is not a sign of Alzheimer's disease. Losing keys is normal. A person with Alzheimer's disease has an uncharacteristic memory loss which makes it difficult to do routine tasks. Forgetting how to balance the checkbook or not knowing how to find the way home could signal the start of dementia.

Most people think Alzheimer's disease is a sudden loss of the mind. Alzheimer's disease progresses slowly. A person who behaves strangely once is probably reacting to stress or some other easily identified factor. If a mild-mannered elderly man gets angry at his wife because she spent too much money he is having a normal reaction to a stressful situation. If the same man loses his temper constantly and begins swearing profusely it is appropriate to suspect dementia.

The person in the early stage may not even be aware of the behavior or may be skilled in disguising the problem. Friends and relatives may overlook the behavior or cover up for the patient because they are embarrassed, frightened, or ignorant.

It is not surprising that this happens. A diagnosis of Alzheimer's disease ends the joking and begins the journey to death. However, the diagnostic process can also have a good end. Many temporary reversible conditions resemble Alzheimer's disease and a thorough examination will reveal those.

— The probability of having the disease increases with age. This is important because the population most likely to become demented is also the fastest growing one.

About 10% of those 65 to 85 years old are affected. Almost 50% of those 85 years old or older have the disease. Today there are 25.5 million Americans 65 years old or older. That number will increase to 67.5 million in 2050 A.D., of which 15 million will be 85 years old or older (U.S. Congress, Office of Technology Assessment, 1987).

Unless a cure for the disease emerges, the number of patients will be overwhelming. Today more than half of the 1.5 million patients in nursing homes have some form of mental illness. Nursing homes expect to double their populations by 2020 A.D., but will fall far short of having enough beds for the anticipated population of demented elderly patients.

All these statistics point toward a need for more respite programs, particularly programs that prolong the time patients can still function in society. As will be seen, early stage patients can function readily in society. This makes early diagnosis all the more imperative.

THE CLINICAL DIAGNOSIS

In the last 5 years many new programs have opened for patients who are diagnosed with Alzheimer's disease. No one should be admitted to an early stage Alzheimer's program until a diagnostic examination is completed. It is possible that a family member or prospective group member may come to a director seeking admission before such an examination. In that case the director should explain the steps in a diagnostic procedure and what to expect. This information should enable the director to do so.

Some states have diagnostic centers which not only administer tests but also counsel families, train health-care professionals, treat patients, and do research. State departments of aging or social services divisions will have a list of centers.

If there is no center close enough, then the patient should make an appointment with a trusted physician. It is likely that the family doctor will refer the patient to a specialist for tests.

The diagnostic procedure consists of three parts:

(a) a medical history,
(b) a medical examination, and
(c) mental tests.

Standard diagnostic criteria have been set by a work group of the U.S. Department of Health and Human Services Task Force on Alzheimer's Disease (McKhann et al., 1984; Tierney et al., 1988).

Medical History

It is preferable for the patient to answer the questions about medical history. If the patient is not coherent then the person most familiar with the patient's history should answer the questions. In any case a caregiver, family member, or friend should come with the patient because the patient may have memory lapses, not understand some questions, or deliberately or unintentionally leave out important information.

The medical history has three parts:

(a) a description of the problem,
(b) a personal health inventory, and
(c) a family medical history.

The goal of the medical history is to determine symptoms, find out whether personal habits or other medical problems have contributed to the condition, and whether family members have had similar illnesses.

The doctor will ask the patient or surrogate to describe the problem. This will include details about when the problem began, what the noticeable changes were, how long the condition has continued, and whether this is the first time it has happened.

The patient will be asked to describe symptoms. The list commonly associated with early stage Alzheimer's disease includes memory loss, mood swings, emotional outbursts, uninhibited behavior, and problems concentrating, performing routine tasks, or using language. The patient will also be asked whether any hallucinations and delusions have occurred; these are a less frequent but possible symptom of early stage Alzheimer's.

The doctor will ask the patient many questions about personal health habits. These will include sleeping patterns, exercise regime, eating habits, and use of alcohol, caffeine, and tobacco. Each of these can affect behavior adversely.

The doctor will discuss hobbies and profession to learn whether the patient has been exposed to chemicals or toxins. Even something as simple as overexposure to glue can trigger behavior changes.

The doctor will want to know what medications the patient has taken. It is best to ask all pharmacists that have supplied medications to provide a list with dosages and frequency of intake. The patient also should mention any nonprescription drugs and be specific about frequency and dosage.

The medication list should be as complete as possible because sometimes nonprescription drugs interact adversely with prescription medications. The doctor will look for drugs that interact adversely, drugs with side effects, and overdosage or overuse of a drug.

The doctor will also ask questions about other problems the

patient has had, particularly within the last year. Among these will be any falls, head injuries, major illnesses, heart attack, or stroke.

Finally, the doctor will take a detailed family history, particularly any record of neurological or mental disease. Heredity affects the probability of disease susceptibility and in some cases is a guarantee a disease will occur.

Medical Examination

The medical examination has three parts:

(a) a clinical checkup,
(b) routine laboratory tests, and
(c) specialized laboratory tests.

The goal is to reveal any other diseases and provide a basic medical profile.

This part of the process can be frightening or humiliating for the patient. At the least, dressing in flimsy gowns, parading through various rooms, and lying on cold tables is embarrassing and uncomfortable. Some patients have a lifelong aversion to having blood samples drawn and others have fears about radiation from X-rays. Even the heartiest patients are reluctant to be encased in machines or prodded with electrodes.

Seeing so many unfamiliar faces and having to be in strange places can be unsettling for a patient who is already having problems coping with daily routines. The problem will be even worse if the patient has to wait long. If possible the tests should be done at a familiar place by people the patient knows and trusts. If not, then technicians should be told in advance if the patient's behavior could be a problem. In any case a definite appointment time should be set and the situation clearly understood by the office staff so that waiting time is kept to a minimum.

It is unrealistic to expect that the patient will believe that the tests won't hurt, won't take a long time, and will result in something good. Most of the patient's normal emotional defenses will be gone or disturbed and the patient is not apt to be calm or rational. Fears about the diagnosis will contribute to the tense situation.

If it is at all possible someone should be with the patient during testing to offer comfort, to be someone to talk with if the wait becomes burdensome, or sometimes simply to see that the patient moves smoothly from site to site.

The clinical checkup shows the doctor any gross motor problems, lung or heart abnormality, muscle tone, and any visible problems such as bruises or lumps.

Routine laboratory tests include checks of the blood and urine. A blood chemistry panel will reveal liver or kidney problems. The blood count and sedimentation rate will disclose infection or the possibility of cancer. The urinalysis is a screen for diabetes and viral infections. Thyroid function and vitamin B_{12} levels will be tested. Both venereal disease and AIDS can cause dementia and if either could be a factor then tests will be done. A chest X-ray will rule out tuberculosis. The doctor may also do other X-rays to determine the patient's general condition. Finally, the doctor may ask for an electrocardiogram, particularly if there is any family history of heart disease.

The specialized tests are more expensive but are useful for identifying conditions with similar symptoms.

The electroencephalogram or EEG monitors the brain's electrical impulses. The technician attaches electrodes to the patient's skull. The process is painless but doesn't look that way; any patient who was already agitated is apt to become even more upset at the prospect of having needles attached, often by a total stranger. It is particularly useful for someone familiar to stand by and reassure the patient until the electrodes are actually operating and the patient can observe that no harm is being done.

An irregular EEG pattern can indicate head injury, trauma, or stroke.

The computerized axial tomography or CAT scan shows abnormalities in the brain such as tumors or clots. It also shows cortical atrophy and enlarged ventricles and sulci, which are typical of Alzheimer's disease, but is not a definite indicator because the pattern can also appear in the brains of people with no cognitive problems.

To conduct a CAT scan, a technician will ask the patient to lie on a table and will then encase the patient's head in a helmet-like machine. The machine will X-ray the patient's head and reveal any abnormalities. A claustrophobic person will not want to take this test and is unlikely even to agree to lie on the table.

Magnetic resonance imaging or MRI tests have the same purpose as CAT scans, but use magnetic beams instead of X-rays to reveal the abnormalities. The MRI chamber is even more confining than the CAT scan helmet and may remind the patient of a coffin. Tests can take up to an hour, during which the machine bombards the patient with sounds resembling those of a jackhammer. This will be a frightening experience for almost any elderly patient and the test should be done only if absolutely necessary. Further, MRI tests are still expensive since the technology is relatively new. If the doctor requires this test it is advisable to discuss the rationale.

Two other possible tests are positron emission tomography or PET scans, and single photon emission computerized tomography, or SPECT. The SPECT test measures blood flow in the brain. A PET scan shows deficits in the temporal and parietal cortex. A normal PET scan is bright and indicates a high level of brain activity. The Alzheimer's disease patient will have a dark PET scan, indicating little brain activity.

Even these sophisticated tests cannot definitively identify Alzheimer's disease. At best the tests are useful measures for identifying other problems and narrowing the diagnosis.

One other test that may be useful is a folic acid test. Chronic alcoholism results in a deficiency of folic acid. This test is more reliable than counting on a patient or caregiver to be truthful about alcoholism, since shame or fear may prohibit full disclosure. Alcoholism can most certainly result in dementia.

Mental Tests

No one single test confirms the presence of Alzheimer's disease; in fact, many scales exist to rate dementia. These clinical and neuropsychological tests were standardized by the Consortium to Establish a Registry for Alzheimer's Disease (CERAD) (Morris et al., 1988). The tests evaluate a patient's memory, logic, abstract reasoning, attention span, and language ability. Some of these tests also evaluate coordination and visuospatial functions.

A thorough discussion of these tests is beyond the scope of this book, but at least one test is so widely used that it bears mention. The Mini-Mental State Examination (Folstein, Folstein, & McHugh, 1975) measures orientation, language, concentration, and immediate and delayed memory. The test is short, simple, and easy to administer and interpret. Some form of the test is used as an admission standard for almost all existing early stage programs (see Appendix C).

DELIRIUM, DEPRESSION, AND DEMENTIA

When the clinical tests are complete the physician can then rule out three conditions often confused with Alzheimer's disease: delirium, depression, and other dementia.

Delirium

Both delirium and Alzheimer's disease involve memory impairment, disorientation, and incoherent behavior including impaired speech. There is a distinct difference, however. Delirium is acute and episodic. People with delirium drift in and out of consciousness. By contrast, Alzheimer's disease is slow and insidious. Its victims maintain a near-constant awareness level.

Delirium can be triggered by fever, toxins, malnutrition, medicine, or a change in metabolism. It can be the result of withdrawal from drugs, a sudden trauma, or even an abrupt change in location if the person is sufficiently fragile, such as the transfer of an elderly nursing home patient. It is possible to correct any of these factors and reverse the progress. Alzheimer's disease cannot be reversed.

Depression

Depression and Alzheimer's disease also have similar symptoms. In both, the patient may be disoriented, restless, or abstracted. The patient may pace or may sleep excessively. The patient is apt to have mood swings, by turns becoming angry, sullen, apathetic, or uncommunicative.

Depression will respond to treatment. It will lessen or disappear altogether with psychotherapy, medication, or sometimes even a change of circumstances such as getting more light, exercising, changing jobs, ending a bad relationship, or simply hearing good news. Alzheimer's disease cannot be cured. Certain behaviors such as agitation, wandering, and sleeplessness can be curtailed with medication, but the disease cannot be reversed. At best it can only be temporarily delayed.

Other Dementia

Dementia is not itself a disease. The term is applied to behaviors and symptoms characteristic of diseases associated with diseased brain tissue. Some dementia are reversible, others irreversible; some progressive, some not; and some temporary, others permanent.

In addition to Alzheimer's disease, the irreversible dementia are multi-infarct or stroke damage, Parkinson's disease, Huntington's disease, Lou Gehrig's disease or amyotrophic lateral sclerosis (ALS), and the rare nerve diseases: Pick's disease, Wilson's disease, and Creutzfeldt-Jakob disease. These diseases are also incurable, but some of the major symptoms can be controlled with medication.

Certain conditions also precipitate the symptoms of dementia. These include, but are not limited to: dehydration, renal failure, reaction to medication, head trauma, viral infections, vitamin deficiencies, chemical poisoning, heart failure, reaction to anesthesia, alcoholism, liver disease, malnutrition, brain tumors, AIDS, syphilis, and hyperglycemia. These conditions can be treated and the dementia reversed. In some cases, such as AIDS, the condition will still be fatal but the dementia's rate of progress can be slowed down.

LEVELS OF DIAGNOSTIC CONFIDENCE

There are three levels of diagnostic confidence (McKhann et al., 1984).

No physician can confirm the definite presence of Alzheimer's disease in a living person. *Definite* Alzheimer's disease is verified only with a histopathologic exam. Although the brain shrinks as much as 40% as the disease progresses, brain weight is not the identifying criterion (Hart & Sample, 1990). The confirming signs are a profusion of neurofibrillary tangles in the temporal and frontal lobes and the hippocampus, neuritic plaques in those areas, and granulovacuolar degeneration in the hippocampus (Hart & Sample, 1990).

In the absence of a biopsy the next level of diagnosis is *probable* Alzheimer's disease. The physician has not identified any other recognizable cause for dementia, but dementia has been evidenced in neuropsychological tests, deficits in at least two cognitive areas and progressive worsening of memory and cognition. Supporting evidence would include a family history of disorders confirmed through biopsy, a normal EEG, progressive cerebral atrophy revealed in a CAT scan or MRI, and a normal lumbar puncture.

The third level is *possible* Alzheimer's disease. The physician has identified other disorders which impair cognition, such as stroke, or atypical symptoms, but has clinical grounds to suspect Alzheimer's disease.

Alzheimer's disease may be ruled out if the onset was apoplectic, there are specific neurological problems such as hemiparesis, or the patient has gait disturbances or early seizures.

DEFINITION OF EARLY STAGE

Lisa Gwyther (1985) is generally credited with describing the disease's course in stages. Variations of her model include anywhere from three to five stages. Broadly speaking, three stages are sufficient to mark major changes.

Stage one is characterized by atypical memory loss, confusion about places, loss of initiative, poor judgment, mood changes, trouble with routine chores, trouble with calculations, and mild aphasia.

Characteristics of *stage two* are greater memory loss, short attention span, problems recognizing people, restlessness, motor problems, weight changes, loss of writing and speech skills including a tendency to repeat things, and wandering.

At *stage three*, the patient does not recognize self or others, loses weight, cannot handle self-care, is incontinent, sleeps most of the time, has seizures, has no language skills, and ultimately has a total shutdown of body functions.

Rigid use of this model would lead to the conclusion that the disease has a uniform pattern when in fact it varies by case. Many so-called stage-one patients, for example, exhibit stage-two symptoms.

The model is merely a general guide for classifying behaviors and symptoms, not a way to identify suitable candidates for an early care program. If a person is labeled stage one but has moderate aphasia, for example, that person is unlikely to be able to take part in group discussions about the disease and hence should not be in the group.

At least one program director addresses the problem by suggesting a variety of designations for patients suitable for an early intervention program: first stage, early stage, early onset, early diagnosis and high functioning (Connee Pence, personal communication, Nov. 17, 1993).

From a purely practical standpoint the most likely candidate for an early intervention program would be one designated as a high-functioning patient. Not all first stage or early diagnosis cases are suitable for day-care programs. Some exhibit severe antisocial behavior or marked speech degeneration. Others have concomitant problems or serious physical limitations. Ultimately, placement in the early intervention program depends entirely on individual assessment, not on arbitrary labels.

CONCLUSION

The layperson lacks the knowledge necessary to detect Alzheimer's disease, but anecdotal information about changes in behavior can indicate a need for a professional diagnosis.

Diagnosis of Alzheimer's disease is largely a process of ruling out other conditions and diseases. Standard tests enable physicians to determine whether factors indicative of early dementia are present.

Statistics reveal an urgent need for the development of early intervention programs. The population needing the programs will burgeon in the next century.

Establishing a Program

2

Certain fundamental subjects must be addressed before launching a program for early stage patients. These include program goals, choice of facility, funding, selection of a board, licensing, and insurance.

Day-care programs provide much needed respite for caregivers. In fact, caregivers have been the primary focus of most respite care programs. First, they enable the caregiver to spend some time away from the patient and to do something other than the incessant work of meeting the patient's physical and emotional needs. Second, such programs usually have a family support component, enabling caregivers to voice their problems in an empathetic setting.

But the early intervention program is different. Unlike mid- to late-stage patients, early stage patients have the ability to name and discuss their disease and the issues it causes in their lives. Therefore, although some attention may be paid to caregivers' concerns, most early intervention groups are focused more on patients' than caregivers' needs.

Program goals reflect this priority. While serving as a social outlet for patients, the groups also offer a range of activities that maximize the patients' remaining skills and build their self-esteem.

Groups can meet in a variety of settings, but the primary goal is to locate a facility that minimizes the patients' physical and emotional discomfort. A secondary consideration is choosing a site which attracts volunteers.

Funding is problematic for existing groups, and almost all participants pay some costs. It is vital to establish a funding base within the first year of operation or else be realistic about the group's longevity.

Depending on where the group meets, and the nature of its activities, it may or may not be necessary to have the program licensed. In fact, most programs are not licensed; they function as social groups which are not subject to the extensive state health care regulations governing day-care programs. Even so, it is preferable to have at least one trained health-care professional providing leadership. Although compassion is a key requirement for volunteers, compassion alone is not the basis for a successful program. The program must have a leader who understands the complex social and medical issues raised by the disease.

All terms for insurance coverage must be spelled out before enrolling patients. Coverage can be arranged through a sponsoring agency, the facility's owners, the patients, or any combination of these.

It is important to examine each of these issues in depth and to tailor a practical program that best fits the local situation and needs.

GOALS

The newly diagnosed Alzheimer's disease patient is at high risk for increased emotional crises. It is common for early stage patients to become withdrawn, isolated, dependent, to reflect a decline in self-worth, and to engage in a greater level of conflict with spouse and family (Krishnan et al., 1988).

About 30 percent of newly diagnosed patients meet the criteria for clinical depression (Teri & Reifler, 1987). In addition, at least one study indicates that 63 percent of newly diagnosed patients self-diagnose as depressed (Burns, Jacoby, & Levy, 1991).

The most common changes in early stages are mild aphasia (language impairment, especially difficulty in finding the right word), inability to handle finances, and a decreased ability to handle complex situations or situations requiring extensive recall.

In younger patients, this diminution of skills most often leads to job termination, and this in turn exacerbates the patient's isolation and dependency. At this stage, patients characteristically deny their limitations and become angry about the situation (Krishnan, 1988).

Basic living skills are not impaired in the early stage. The patient is capable of self-care, not incontinent, and can make choices about activities. However, many newly diagnosed patients slip rapidly into deep depression and begin to neglect these basic functions (Krishnan, 1988).

In turn, caregivers experience and report high stress levels even in early stages (Stevenson, 1990). Many experience such concerns as fear that the disease is hereditary, frustration at the breakdown of normal communication patterns, loss and grief, anger at not being in control, and guilt when or if negative feelings about the patient arise.

It is important to decrease this stress (Harper & Lund, 1990). The person who denies or represses emotions in the beginning will probably not be able to cope as the situation gets worse. The painful emotions will intensify and the caregiver may well lose all empathy for the patient. Respite care allows the caregiver a chance to step back and take a look at the situation while remaining assured that the patient is receiving proper care (Strang & Neufeld, 1990).

Until the late 1980s, the caregiver had few options. Respite workers could be hired to come to the home while caregivers took vacations or short trips. Some Alzheimer's Association chapters offered caregiver support groups. Or caregivers could seek out a day-care program for mid- to late-stage patients. These options, however, offered nothing for the early stage patient.

While the caregiver might be uncomfortable in leaving the early stage patient at home alone, and thus be relieved by hiring a respite worker, the patient is likely to have a different view. Already wary of changes in routine, the patient is apt to view the respite worker as an unwelcome intruder or a surrogate babysitter, symbolizing the deterioration the patient is most likely not yet ready to accept. The patient will at best feel denigrated and at worst react with hostility toward the stranger.

Similarly, programs for mid- to late-stage patients are not suitable for early stage patients. Such programs do not offer adequate social challenge, physical activity, or mental stimulation for early stage patients.

In September 1988 the Lexington/Bluegrass, Kentucky, chapter of the Alzheimer's Association launched "The Lunch Bunch," a pilot program for people with mild memory impairment. The program received an award at the 1989 national Alzheimer's Association meeting, and the national association noted both the dearth of other programs and the necessity for them.

Between 1988 and 1993 at least 18 other early stage programs were started (Wylie, 1993a). The Greater San Francisco Bay Area chapter of the Alzheimer's Association intends to set up several pilot programs and has therefore done a study of known programs to find out what has worked elsewhere. Information about such programs is sketchy.

The Bay Area chapter gleaned its information from program brochures, telephone calls to program directors, unpublished memos, and responses to a national Alzheimer's Association 1990 survey of support groups (see Appendix A for a list of these support groups).

A limited amount of printed material about support groups is also available (Drickamer & Lachs, 1991; Goldstein, 1991; and Zgola & Coulter, 1988).

A consistent, if limited and non-empirical, portrait of the rationale and goals for early stage support groups emerges from these materials.

Basically, three goals emerge from literature describing existing programs: (a) decrease the patient's loneliness, (b) increase the patient's self-esteem, and (c) maximize the patient's remaining physical, mental, and social skills.

Some groups also have a fourth goal—to educate the patient about the problems and process of the disease. However, some support groups do not even speak about the disease; they function purely as social clubs.

As can clearly be seen, these goals address the unique problems of early stage diagnosis: depression, aphasia, and decreased functioning, leading to job loss.

These goals are addressed in a variety of settings and with a variety of therapeutic approaches. Some programs articulate theoretical foundations in print. For example, The Adult Activities Center, in Costa Mesa, California, utilizes milieu therapy (Prather, 1993), while Holland Community Hospital in Holland, Michigan, applies the focus group model (Yalom, 1983). These approaches shall be discussed in detail in the chapter on programming and activities (see Chapter 7).

Some controversy exists as to whether early stage patients should be told the diagnosis (Drickamer & Lachs, 1991). Patients and caregivers are almost invariably devastated by the initial diagnosis, and some programs never mention the disease. Others indicate that disclosure to the patient is not only useful in achieving the three goals but in fact is also essential to program structure (Cooper, 1984; Maves & Schulz, 1985).

Patients who are aware of the diagnosis may not at first articulate issues but, in a tolerant and accepting therapeutic situation, can begin to explore the impact of the disease on their lives and the lives of others (Cooper, 1984).

A number of therapeutic approaches can be used to draw out patients and get them to discuss their issues. Among these are the feeling group model (Van Wylen & Dykema-Lamse, 1990), which focuses on the impact the disease has on the patients' lives. This model will be discussed in depth in the chapter on program structure (see Chapter 7).

Again, the underlying aim of the process is to increase the patients' self-esteem and independence. All group leaders are in agreement that a successful program should include physical exercise. Exercise does not cure Alzheimer's disease, but does increase the patient's well-being through cardiovascular and emotional stimulation (Blair, Brill, & Kohl, 1989; Lindemuth & Moose, 1990). The patient's muscular degeneration is retarded and depression lessened by regular physical stimulation. Physical activities reported by existing groups range from basic conditioning exercises to dancing, golf, and baseball.

In addition to providing a therapeutic community and physical conditioning, most groups offer one or more activities designed to emphasize the patient's continuing role in the larger society. Lunches together at restaurants, visits to museums and other community sites, and picnics at local parks all remind patients that their world is still broad enough to include the activities everyone else enjoys. Last, many groups provide patients a chance to do volunteer work at local agencies, thus reinforcing the concept that they still have a contribution to make to society.

Specific activities and analysis of the relative success and failure of each appears in subsequent chapters.

Given the goals and activities of early stage groups, it is essential that participants meet four criteria: 1) They must be continent; 2) They must not wander or be agitated; 3) They must be able to communicate, and preferably be able to name and discuss their disease; and 4) They must be able to take part in physical activity.

Little has been discussed to date about the effect of accepting patients with marginal behavior, but a homogeneous grouping is more conducive to achieving therapeutic goals (Clemmer, 1992). High-functioning patients tend to withdraw when placed with those less capable, while lower-functioning patients become agitated when unable to keep up with the group. A careful health screening (see Appendix B) can enable group leaders to screen out people who do not fit the group's purposes.

Care should be taken in the intake assessment. Group leaders should screen patients themselves rather than relying exclusively on high scores on the Mini-Mental Status Exam or on caregivers' observations.

In summary:

- The early stage program focuses more on patients than on caregivers.
- Participants are most likely to succeed if they are told their diagnosis.
- The primary goal of group process is to increase participants' self-esteem.
- Group activities should focus on patients' continuing role in society.
- Every program should include an exercise component.
- High-functioning and low-functioning patients should not be in the same group.
- Self-evalulation is important in selection of group members.

FACILITY

At least two factors are important in facility choice: (a) the physical restrictions of the patients, and (b) the likelihood of encouraging volunteer involvement.

Most respite programs are housed in churches, synagogues or senior centers (Brookdale Foundation, 1987). Other groups meet in hospitals or public facilities such as schools.

Uniquely, "The Lunch Bunch," in Kentucky, met exclusively in homes "because of patient sensitivity to institutions" (Wylie, 1993a).

Choosing a safe and familiar site in a residential neighborhood—a church or a synagogue—gives the program an immediate, established, and visible presence in the community. Potential clients and volunteers are readily drawn to the site.

A major factor is that neither clients nor volunteers need worry about transportation to a remote or unsafe area. Church or synagogue members will, as well, be apt to support the program as an extension of their religious commitment (Brookdale Foundation, 1987). Senior centers are a natural hub for volunteers, many looking for a worthy activity to add to their day.

Less conducive to volunteer involvement are the programs conducted in hospitals and other institutional settings. For example, a clinical social worker at the Neuropsychiatric Institute, Los Angeles, California, conducts group therapy for newly diagnosed patients, but she notes that the group has provoked "little interest among interns" and has no outside volunteers or support program (Wylie, 1993a).

Religious bodies and senior centers are also better prepared to deal with such potentially troubling issues as security measures, janitorial services, and insurance coverage for on-site programs. It is not difficult to write the program into existing policies and procedures. Groups attempting to handle such issues without the help of a sponsoring agency may find that both high expense and time needed are well beyond the means of the group. However, simply because the facility is apt to draw volunteers is not sufficient reason to use it. If it does not meet the minimal standards for patients' safety and comfort, other options should be considered.

The overall goal of site selection is to obtain the facility that best minimizes the patients' anxiety about impairment. Various designs aid this process (Perlmuter, Tenney, & Smith, 1980; Zarit, Zarit, & Reeves, 1982).

At least four criteria are mandatory (Brawley, 1992).

1. The facility is safe and secure. The staff can monitor patients at all times.
2. The facility does not have a confusing design or a complex decorating scheme.
3. The facility offers space for stimulating activities but does not contain symbols of institutionalization such as nurses' stations and beds.
4. The site is comfortable, clean, well-lighted, attractive, and nurturing to the patients.

Many religious facilities have numerous side passages, corridors, and small rooms. This maze is undesirable because staff cannot see patients at all times. A self-contained setting, such as a social hall with bathrooms and a kitchen, is preferable, but with these caveats: (a) all doors in the main hall must be visible, and (b) should be locked at all times. If the kitchen has a back exit it should be locked at all times.

This kind of security not only precludes the possibility of patients wandering, but also secludes the area from other activities in the building. Passersby will not be able to enter the locked area, thus eliminating distractions which have the potential to agitate patients. Obviously, a clear arrangement should be made with the facility's owners about exclusive use of the area during the respite program.

There is no reason to choose a facility that is dingy, shabby, dirty, or depressing. Religious institutions, senior centers, and public buildings are generally clean, but avoid choosing such a site if furnishings are shabby, paint is dingy, or the building feels dark and depressing.

Obviously, patients and staff simply will not feel good about coming to the program if it is held in a shabby, dirty setting. But the requirements for light, color, and other design details are not simply aesthetic preferences.

Almost all elderly patients have minor to severe levels of vision impairment. Color and depth perception are reduced in the aging process. The eye's lens changes as it ages, and over time everything takes on a yellow-brown cast.

Aging people cannot distinguish shades and tones; that is, they often have trouble recognizing such colors as mauve and pale blue. While these colors may seem soothing to designers, in fact they exacerbate the patient's problems. Clear colors with strong contrasts are preferable. In particular, the elderly patient needs to be in an area where there is a sharp contrast between the floors, walls, and doors (Altman, 1986). This sets spatial boundaries clearly, reduces the risk of falls, and eliminates confusion about how and where to move about.

In addition, floors and walls should be in contrasting mono-tones, without borders or trim. Rugs and vinyl with patterns and walls with borders disrupt depth perception. Some patients become distracted and pick endlessly at the patterns and de-signs.

Research indicates that the popular practice of color-coding of rooms or corridors—red indicating a bathroom door, blue a bed-room—is virtually worthless as an environmental clue (Brawley, 1992). This is because mentally impaired older people generally rely on smell and tactile clues to orient themselves. It is true that the sense of smell also decreases with age, but correspondingly, certain smells become guideposts associated with specific places or events. For example, freshly cut grass may trigger a desire to take a walk, or baking cookies may draw the person to the kitchen.

Early research suggested that religious institutions, designed as places to encourage meditation and quiet, had a calming ef-fect on patients (Brookdale Foundation, 1987). But such facilities can also have the opposite impact. If the building is shadowy and has dim lighting, it will confuse and disturb the patient. The patient will be most comfortable in a well lit area where boundaries are clear, shapes and forms are easily recognized for what they are, and there are no surprises hidden in the dimness.

There will not necessarily be choices in the color schemes at the chosen facility, but at least certain guidelines should be met. It is best to avoid a place with patterned carpets or fussy wallpaper, for example.

Another major design consideration is acoustics. In addition to sight, hearing diminishes with age. Background noises become more distracting, interfere with communication, and often agitate the elderly.

While a sanctuary might have excellent acoustics, the better to show off a choir's musical skills, the other rooms in religious facilities often have poor or no acoustic provisions. It is important to see how sound works in the chosen rooms.

At minimum, the chosen facility should be carpeted; this will absorb some sound. Other items, such as furniture, plants, paintings, and other artworks also improve acoustics. However, if these objects are themselves distracting, such as an elaborate wall hanging that interferes with depth perception, then the good done in reducing noise is offset by the agitation felt by the patient.

It is important, therefore, to check the space to see which items are permanently displayed and whether these add to or detract from the overall setting.

Furniture should be chosen with care. Ergonomic factors are a key consideration in choosing furniture. Choose chairs that allow the patient's feet to touch the floor. High chairs are not suitable because the patient's feet will dangle and will soon become numb, cold, or filled with fluid. If a chair is too wide or deep, the patient will slump, putting pressure on organs and precipitating incontinence (Lieb, 1982). Recliners are unsuitable because they put too much pressure on the buttocks.

In general, chairs upholstered in textured fabrics are preferable. These give the patients something comfortable to touch. Oilcloth or vinyl is easier to clean, but can be slippery, and is sensually uninviting.

The site should contain at least one table, preferably a round one so that everyone is able to see everyone else during activities. The table will be the place where group members sit to talk with each other, eat, and look at photographs. Many older patients will be reminded of happy times spent at their own kitchen tables.

Heavy, bulky furniture is undesirable. Staff members and patients should be able to move furniture with minimum effort. If chairs and other furniture are lined up in rows against the walls, the setting will resemble an institution and patients could become agitated. Chairs should be grouped in informal seating arrangements much as they would be in a home.

However, furniture that will tip or fall easily should also be avoided. Pole lamps without a heavy base, many kinds of folding chairs, pedestal tables, and similar items are decorative and light, but unstable. Any item of furniture should be able to bear a patient's weight without tipping or shaking.

Finally, it is important to choose a facility where the temperature can be controlled. Patients will not necessarily be able to judge their own needs. The leader must make certain that rooms are kept at comfortable levels at all times, since temperatures can vary with sunlight or the opening of windows. Rooms that are too hot or too cold, drafty, have poor air circulation, or where there is no control of temperature should be avoided.

To sum up, these are major considerations in site choice:

- A building in a safe residential neighborhood will draw volunteers.
- A self-contained site, such as a recreation center with bathroom and kitchen, is the ideal site. Avoid mazes of rooms and areas where doors cannot be seen.
- Choose a site with good lighting. Avoid shadowy rooms and dim lighting.
- Choose a room with sharp color contrasts. The elderly cannot distinguish shades and tones.
- The floors should be carpeted with a monotone carpet.
- The walls should not have borders or elaborately designed wallpaper.
- Choose a site with acoustics designed to reduce noise.
- The ideal furniture will include ergonomically designed, textured chairs, and at least one large round table.
- Furniture should be light enough to move with ease but so stable that it will not tip over if full body weight is applied.
- Choose a site where the leader controls the temperature.

The ideal site will compensate for participants' losses, but need not be a sterile institutional setting nor a room distinguished only by its collection of mismatched castoffs. Simplicity and good ergonomic and acoustical design at the chosen site will go a long way toward making the program a success.

FUNDING

Nearly all groups report problems with funding. Groups rely heavily on lay volunteer labor, although both the Eastern Massachusetts, and Baltimore, Maryland, programs are led by unpaid professionals. In most other cases the professionals who serve as directors work on-site anywhere from four hours a month (Rochester, NY) to four days a week (San Diego, CA). Salaries, although generally the major part of a group's budget, are low on the professional scale, and benefits are minimal or not offered. In reality, some directors work many additional unpaid hours, doing such tasks as recruiting new members, testing them, counseling family members, and publicizing the program in the community.

If the facility is licensed as a day-care program by the state, then a certain amount of government support is available. However, such groups must pay licensing fees, hire staff who meet state requirements, and find a facility that fits strict state regulations. The costs usually offsets the revenue. The San Diego Morning Out Club, which has four sites, pays $600 per site for license fees alone.

Programs sponsored by medical centers, such as the one in Granada Hills, California, can bill health insurance for the services of psychologists and speech therapists. But location in a medical facility is not an assurance of survival. The program in Los Angeles, now in its third year, "has a doubtful future: re budget cuts," according to its director (Wylie, 1993a). The Granada Hills program began in 1993 and has yet to be evaluated in future budgets or under pending health care reforms.

More than half of the programs rely on grants. In general, programs that rely on grants stand little chance of survival. Grants are generally time-limited and many are renewable only if the program can show clear evidence of finding ongoing supplemental support.

Unfortunately, group leaders have a tendency to avoid these realities and to conduct the program as if the first flush of financial security were permanent. The other unfortunate reality is that neither the director nor volunteers usually have the time or the ability to apply for funding from other sources.

It is essential that grant-funded programs address this reality from the onset. Any program should have at least six months' funds in reserve at all times. Having a strong board of directors who either take on the task of fund-raising, or hiring a person to do development, is essential for program survival.

In general, it is a good idea to complement grant funding with a mix of other fund-raising options. These can range from direct mail solicitation to corporate appeals to specific fund-raising events such as raffles and dinners. In the case of both grant and corporate fund-raising, it is not enough to offer a program with good intentions. At the least, be prepared to state the program's objectives, to present its charter, list of board members and operating budget, and to explain what unique services the program offers to the local community. Neither corporate executives nor grant boards have the time or interest to waste on poorly prepared proposals and most will not offer a second hearing.

The first early intervention program, the Kentucky Lunch Bunch, was funded by a Robert Wood Johnson grant. In 1992 when the grant ran out, the program was discontinued, "due to lack of time and money" (Wylie, 1993a).

By contrast, the Ann Arbor, Michigan, Early Stage Memory Loss Program, which was also originally funded by grant, is now funded by the South Central Michigan Chapter of the Alzheimer's Association. The comprehensive program includes an in-home screening by a social worker and a support group for caregivers.

In general, those groups that affiliate with Alzheimer's associations seem to be most successful in getting grants.

For example, San Diego's Morning Out Club, sponsored by the San Diego Chapter of the Alzheimer's Association, is doing a three-year study comparing the merits of various program strategies at the Club's four locations.

In more than half the groups, participants pay a minimal fee, $10 to $35 per half-day session. Programs which charge fees note that prices have been raised in the past two years, and some programs which did not charge fees on inception now do so.

In summary, these are funding options:

- State fees as a licensed day-care center.
- Grants.
- Health insurance billing under a medical center's sponsorship.
- Patient fees or donations.
- Corporate appeals.
- Fund-raising events.
- Affiliation with an Alzheimer's Association or other sponsoring agency.

Each option has limitations which should be considered carefully. A key in stable funding is having a strong board of directors whose top priority is fund-raising. Another key is direct confrontation with the issues of ongoing funding; grants are time-limited and often contingent on matching funding. Other options should be explored, but do not base the funding appeals on the good intentions of the program; provide hard data. Patient fees must be raised periodically to reflect economic realities. Health insurance coverage is in transition and is not a guarantee of financial success.

CHOOSING A BOARD OF DIRECTORS

The board of directors is responsible for the administration of the program. Its members ensure compliance with laws and safety regulations, oversee the fiscal health of the program, set policy, and monitor the services provided.

Many boards have members who are nothing more than tokens. They seldom or never attend meetings, provide no services, and sometimes do not even know, understand, or agree with the program's goals. Avoid token board members.

Board members should be vitally interested in the program and actively involved in ensuring its place in the community. It is wisest to choose a board of skilled professionals whose expertise will further the program's goals. At minimum, the board should include an attorney, a business manager, a public relations or marketing professional, a personnel director, a social services worker, and at least one person with knowledge of Alzheimer's disease and patients' needs. Some boards may also wish to have at least one caregiver as a member, or at the least, ask a caregiver to serve as advisor to the board.

It may also be desirable to appoint an advisory board. Generally the members of such a group are chosen for their ability to perform certain vital functions such as fund-raising or publlc relations.

In both cases, it is advisable to appoint board members who represent the ethnic and economic makeup of the community. This will be mandatory if the group receives government funding.

Although it should be obvious, members should have had personal experience with Alzheimer's disease patients; some empathy is a vital requirement for board membership.

Each group should have a set of written documents including, but not limited to, bylaws, personnel policies, list of board members, description of board duties, and budget information. If the group is a nonprofit organization the board needs to have a copy of all required incorporation documents and quarterly reports.

The board should establish policies about insurance, transportation, medication, and plans for disasters.

Since volunteers provide most of the programs' services, it is a good idea to provide written descriptions of what is expected of volunteers. This should include some requirement for supervised training in the issues that arise in the care of Alzheimer's patients.

In sum:

• Do not appoint token board members.
• Appoint a board that represents the ethnic and economic makeup of the community.

- Appoint a board with diverse professional skills.
- Each board member should have personal experience with Alzheimer's disease patients.
- Policies and procedures should be in writing, particularly requirements for volunteers.

LICENSING

Some programs can be licensed as adult day-care centers. Each state has its own regulations and fees for licensing. In general, the programs that are licensed are based on a medical care model; that is, the programs are managed and supervised by trained medical personnel, minimal or no attention is paid to social activities, and the program is usually associated with a hospital or geriatrics center. Often the aim is to prepare patients for entry into a day-care program for advanced stage patients, or a residential program.

In most states, requirements for obtaining a day-care license are stringent and include everything from specific facility design to extensive paperwork for each patient. Staff must have special licenses and even volunteers must meet certain criteria. These standards are monitored by either the state department of health services or the state social services division, and such programs are reviewed annually for recertification.

Most programs will find that certification is unnecessary and unduly expensive. Most programs are not licensed. Instead the programs function as informal social clubs or programs of the local Alzheimer's Association.

Regardless of certification status, each program must meet fire and safety standards. If the program is held in a local church or school, it is not sufficient to assume that the facility's fire codes will suffice for the new program. The board must contact the fire marshal and ask for an inspection and release before holding the program.

In sum:

- Some programs can be licensed as day-care centers, but must meet strict state standards and pay all applicable licensing fees.
- Most programs are not licensed.
- All programs must meet fire and safety standards before beginning operation.

INSURANCE

Each program must be certain that liability insurance is provided for both personnel and board. In cases where professionals such as nurses are involved, the individuals must have malpractice coverage.

The board should consider all potential situations, including transportation coverage, accidents at the facility, disaster coverage, and even the improbable but possible results of adverse reaction to foods at public sites.

In most instances the patients will also have personal medical insurance. The director should have a file with this information about each patient, including emergency contacts, list of preferred medical facilities, emergency insurance authorization numbers, and any other information needed in the event of emergency care. If the emergency contact is not going to be readily available, the director should also have authorization to have the patient receive emergency care. The director should not rely on the patient having a medical card readily available; the file should include information sufficient for an admission without a card.

If a program is licensed as a day-care center it will receive some state funding for each participant, although seldom enough to offset licensing costs. Medicare does not provide coverage for such programs but some state Medicaid programs do allocate funds for day care.

To review:

- Board and personnel must have liability insurance.
- The director should keep a file with information about each patient's medical insurance.
- Some state health-care insurance is available for licensed day-care centers.

CONCLUSION

Many issues must be resolved before a program begins operation. While empathy and good intentions are basic for program planning, they are insufficient for success.

More important are long-range financial planning, careful selection of a skilled board, and knowledge of community and state regulations. It is also important to articulate program goals, expectations for personnel and volunteers, and board responsibilities.

No program need settle for second-rate facilities, thoughtless program management, or insufficient funding. Careful advance planning is the key to success.

Choosing Staff

3

The size and professional credentials of staff will depend upon the size and purpose of the program. However, anyone working with early stage patients will need compassion, humor, patience, and initiative. Care of Alzheimer's patients, even in the early stage, is labor-intensive and emotionally demanding.

Early intervention programs rely heavily on volunteers. Unlike most other situations where volunteers do whatever needs to be done, the volunteer in an early intervention program does a specific task and needs special training. The volunteer should be treated like a paid staff member in terms of training, responsibilities, and accountability.

The purpose of staff training is to impart information, clarify the program goals and philosophy, and assess staff members' attitudes and skill levels.

SIZE AND CREDENTIALS OF STAFF

Each patient will need extensive attention, whether in actual physical help with doing activities or simply in meaningful personal interactions. The average staff-to-participant ratio is one to three, although if patients are very highly skilled the ratio can be as high as one to five (Lindemann, Corby, Downing, & Sanborn, 1991). Most programs have only two or three staff members and often only one is a professional.

In all cases, it is essential that a minimum of two staff members be present at all times. A crisis or even a minor problem can demand the director's full attention at any time and it is not acceptable to leave the patients alone for even a short time.

The kind of staff depends upon the kinds of services offered. For example, the Granada Hills Community Hospital in Granada Hills, California, is a medical-based program including speech therapy and psychological counseling. Staff members include a gerontologist, psychologist, speech therapist, occupational therapist, and exercise physiologist (Wylie, 1993a).

By contrast, the Friends Club of Washington, D.C., relies on volunteers. Each patient has a companion volunteer and there are also two staff members (Tully & Turner, 1992).

When deciding how many people to hire and what their credentials should be, these points should be kept in mind:

- A minimum of two people should be on-site at all times.
- The ideal ratio of staff to patient is one to three, but in very high functioning groups, it can be as high as one to five.
- Professional credentials will depend upon the program's goals. Some programs can succeed with volunteers.

DIRECTOR

Often the program director is the only paid staff member and the only professional directly involved with the program. However, the director is generally a part-time employee, with many responsibilities but few or no benefits, and a low salary.

It is important for the board to consider both factors when interviewing candidates for the job. The director has primary responsibility for the administration and success of the program and should be highly qualified in many areas. However, the job demands are unusually high for low financial and professional returns, so the candidate must also genuinely love the work and be willing to accept the job's demands and limitations.

Any candidate who is unrealistic about salary raises, job requirements, or time commitments should be eliminated regardless of qualifications.

Because much of the burden of evaluating patients and dealing with families will be the director's responsibility, the director should be a trained gerontologist, social worker, mental health professional, or any other professional with extensive knowledge of aging issues.

In interviewing candidates, the board should establish the person's general knowledge of aging and specific knowledge of Alzheimer's disease. Occasionally a skilled layperson may be able to direct a program, but only those with direct experience with patients should be considered.

At a minimum, the director must understand how to keep records, track medication, respond to medical emergencies, and train and supervise other staff members including volunteers.

In addition, the director must be skilled in dealing with the public. The director will have many responsibilities involving extensive public contact including marketing the program, grant writing, family counseling, and reporting to the board on a regular basis.

It is necessary for the director and the board to be in accord about program goals and management. The hours of operation, fee schedules, and other basic procedures should all be specified in writing. All legal matters such as fire clearances, nonprofit status, and licenses should be thoroughly reviewed and a procedure established for updates. Further, the chain of authority should be clearly specified so that any disputes or problems can be speedily resolved.

Each employee should have a formal contract specifying responsibilities, salary, personnel policies, and in the unlikely event it is needed, the mediation process. Often the director will be the only paid staff member. However, unpaid staff members and volunteers should have written job descriptions.

The director's contract should include a provision for continuing education. Information about Alzheimer's disease changes rapidly and the director should be encouraged to stay updated. Attending educational forums is a practical way to exchange experiences and information. It is also emotionally beneficial for directors to interact with peers.

The contract should include provisions for vacation and respite time and the time frames should be monitored and enforced by the board. Nonprofit managers are particularly prone to skipping vacations or failing to schedule one until forced to do so. The best option is to choose mutually agreeable dates when the program will not be affected.

The board's personnel committee should evaluate the director on a regular basis, and not less than once a year. Insofar as is possible without interfering with the program, board members should come on-site occasionally to observe the director at work. The evaluation should be written and the director should be given a chance to respond in writing.

Usually the director is responsible for supervising other staff and volunteers and for any terminations. However, no personnel decisions should be final without the approval of the board. This safeguards against the possibility of arbitrary action by a director. Occasionally a board may choose to be entirely responsible for all personnel matters including overseeing volunteers.

The ideal director is:

• Familiar with aging and Alzheimer's disease.
• Aware of the extensive demands of the job and willing to accept the pay and responsibilities.
• Aware of the program's goals and procedures.

ASSISTANT DIRECTOR

The assistant director can be a trained professional, a student in a relevant field, or a committed volunteer. The assistant director may have less training than the director, but should have previous experience with patients and training in aging and Alzheimer's disease.

The assistant director is in charge if the director is unexpectedly ill or absent. This means the assistant director should be familiar with the same procedures and management issues as the director and prepared to run the program for a short time. However, the assistant director should not attempt to conduct a regular session unless at least one volunteer is also present. As mentioned, an emergency could require the assistant director's entire attention and patients should not be left alone, even briefly. The assistant director should have enough initiative to cancel a session if unprepared or if another person is not present.

Volunteers usually handle logistical details in larger programs, but in smaller ones, the assistant director may be the one who greets patients when they arrive, drives them to various activities, supervises crafts or other activities, or takes patients to the toilet.

The assistant director usually has a great deal of contact with families at the program site. The more often the family members see the assistant director the more likely they are to talk about the patient or their issues. The assistant director should have some counseling skills and should be able to report any relevant information to the director.

The director and assistant director should meet weekly, possibly at the end of each week's session, to discuss issues and make plans for the next session.

It is important that the assistant director and the director like each other and work together well. Early stage patients are susceptible to emotional tension and are apt to pick up on any staff conflicts regardless of how quiet or subtle these may be.

However, it is acceptable, and even desirable, if the director and assistant director have different personalities. As long as the styles are complementary and not antagonistic, the patients will benefit from working with people who see a situation from many perspectives.

The ideal assistant director is:

- Trained in aging and Alzheimer's disease.
- Able to do the director's job in the event of an emergency or capable of canceling the program.
- Skilled at listening to families and reporting relevant information to the director.
- Compatible with the director.

VOLUNTEERS

However well-meaning the offer, it is not advisable to accept a patient's caregiver as a volunteer. The caregiver gets no respite and the patient is likely to be inhibited in the presence of the caregiver.

Similarly, it is inadvisable to have newly bereaved caregivers serve as volunteers. The emotional traumas are too fresh and it is too easy for such a volunteer to transfer inappropriate feelings to the situation.

Volunteers can come from a variety of settings: churches and synagogues, senior centers, community agencies, and colleges. In the case of early care programs, it is common for volunteers to come from the agency or group sponsoring the program (Brookdale Foundation, 1987).

All volunteers must have a rudimentary knowledge of aging and Alzheimer's disease. It is preferable that they have direct experience with the aging.

The volunteer for the early care program must possess special skills needed for interacting with the patients. The volunteers must genuinely enjoy close personal interactions, be patient and soft-spoken, and be able to assess unusual situations quickly and take necessary action.

It is important that volunteers perceive themselves as part of a team. Paid staff and volunteers should meet regularly, at least monthly, to discuss the program, any issues that arise, and other important matters.

The volunteer in an early care program should be assigned specific tasks for each meeting. One might be a driver, another collect the money for meals out, and a third arrange the seating at the restaurant.

Volunteers should be placed around the room so that the staff-to-patient ratio is constant at all times. It will be up to each staff to decide whether a particular volunteer shall be the partner of a particular client throughout the program, or whether volunteers work with a different client each week.

Volunteers should:

• Not be family members or newly bereaved caregivers.
• Be trained in aging and Alzheimer's disease.
• Be treated like part of a professional team.
• Assigned specific duties.

TRAINING

All staff, including volunteers, need to meet for training sessions before the program begins. Training sessions should be a minimum of a half day and can last as long as a week. The training session rather than the actual program is the place to test attitudes, skill levels, morale, and knowledge.

Training has three purposes: (a) to impart information, (b) to clarify the philosophy and goals of the program, and (c) to test the skills and reactions of staff members in simulated scenarios.

Knowledge

All staff members should have been pre-screened and should have a general knowledge of aging and some specific knowledge of Alzheimer's disease.

The director should prepare a pretest and administer it at the beginning of training. No one will be required to reveal test results but the group will discuss the answers. The purpose of the test is to bring all staff members up to the same level of knowledge.

A typical true–false test might contain these questions:

1. All old people are going to get Alzheimer's disease. *(False)*
2. Senility and Alzheimer's disease are the same thing. *(False)*
3. Alzheimer's disease is progressive, irreversible, and incurable. *(True)*
4. Doctors can tell if a person has Alzheimer's disease by giving an MRI. *(False)*
5. Cooking in aluminum pots causes Alzheimer's disease. *(False)*
6. People with Alzheimer's disease don't remember anything. *(False)*
7. Exercise and diet are important if a person has Alzheimer's disease. *(True)*
8. A person can have Alzheimer's disease for more than 20 years. *(True)*
9. Everybody with Alzheimer's disease is in a nursing home. *(False)*

The pretest is designed to dispel widespread misconceptions such as the popular but erroneous belief that using aluminum pots causes the disease. The pretest also uncovers less common errors such as the belief that a doctor can make a definite diagnosis with sophisticated tests such as the MRI or CAT scan.

The pretest also reveals staff members' attitudes about the people who have the disease. Some staff members may not know that early care patients can do most activities that normal people can do, or that the disease can occur in middle age.

This part of the training is the appropriate time to pass out handouts and reading lists or to have a doctor or other specialist such as a social worker give a lecture on the disease and its impact.

Any supplemental materials and lectures should be equally weighted with factual matter and information about the social and personal impacts of the disease. The ideal training will instill empathy as well as knowledge.

Simulations

The experiential training has two parts: (a) simulation of being an elderly person, and (b) typical program scenarios.

A number of exercises will help staff members understand what it feels like to be old. Completing the simulations will enable the staff members to know first-hand about the patients' physical limitations and to understand more clearly how to deal with patients in light of those limitations.

These are typical problems of the elderly and ways to simulate the experience:

1. *Blurred vision.* Wear a pair of glasses smeared with Vaseline. Try to walk, do daily tasks, or see another person's face.

2. *Loss of peripheral vision.* Block off side vision by holding the hands up alongside the eyes. Try to determine what the person standing alongside is doing.

3. *Impaired memory.* Have someone read a list of unfamiliar words rapidly. Then try to repeat the list accurately.

4. *Sensitivity to shouting.* Have someone shout constantly about what is to be done next. Observe how quickly pulse increases, tension mounts, and orders become confusing.

This is the time to stress communication techniques such as the need to speak slowly and clearly in a low, calm voice and to repeat sentences if necessary, to look the patient directly in the eye when speaking, to minimize distractions, and to be patient and kind if the person does not understand or is confused.

Other simulations are designed to test staff members' reactions and attitudes to typical day-care scenarios. Patient behavior will be discussed in greater detail in another chapter (see Chapter 6), but among behaviors that can create difficulty are stubbornness, agitation, the urgent need to toilet, failure to remember words, anger, and withdrawal.

First the director or staff trainer will present the scenario, usually in writing so that everyone will know exactly what is happening.

Here is a typical scenario:

> Jim, 72, does not want to work on the crafts project. He says only children play with paints. He won't even sit at the table with the other patients. He keeps trying to leave the room and snaps at any staff member who approaches him.

Next the trainer will ask the group to act out the situation and to think about how it feels to confront the problem. The person who is in the role of Jim should be as uncooperative as possible, while other staff members should try whatever it seems it will take to get Jim to stop being stubborn.

Various responses should emerge. One staff member will try to get Jim to come to the table and watch everyone else paint. Another will want to lead Jim to the table, put a brush in Jim's hand, and attempt to guide the brushstrokes. A third will sit down with Jim away from the group and have a drink and a conversation with Jim. A fourth will call Jim's wife and tell her to come take Jim home.

The group will then write down all the responses and any others that could have been tried. Together the group will evaluate each response and determine why it worked or did not (Lindemann et al., 1991).

Rather than embarrass someone who has done the wrong thing, the director can use the group process to emphasize the most appropriate response to behavior problems. It is especially important to do this in a simulation rather than on the job, where staff and patients would both be hurt by the confrontation.

This is time when staff members can best talk about emotional responses to the scenarios. One staff member may be frightened by anger, for example, while another may respond to anger with anger.

Staff members will also learn whether they are motivated by pity, which is inappropriate, or if their attitudes are patronizing, which is also inappropriate. Again, assessing the situation in a group setting is the ideal way to avoid singling out individuals while eliminating undesirable attitudes.

Goals

As the staff works through the exercises and simulations the group should begin to bond. Only when that level of group trust is reached is it appropriate to approach the philosophical issues of goals

In the absence of experiential knowledge goals are often little more than idealistic proclamations. It is one thing to declare that the major goal of the program is to treat each individual with dignity. It is another to say the same thing after having become angry during a simulated session with a stubborn client.

Realistic goals should take into account the limits of the staff and the likelihood of unforeseen circumstances disrupting even the most careful plans. Obviously it is a good idea to strive for dignity and respect, but at some point everyone will confront negative emotions and difficult situations.

In summary, the training program has many goals.

- It educates staff members about basic facts but also about attitudes and emotions.
- It provides a chance for experiential learning designed to screen out potential problems in the actual program.
- It prepares staff members to be realistic about what a program can accomplish.

CONCLUSION

Attitude is as important as skills in choosing a staff for an early stage program. Each person, including volunteers, should have a detailed written statement of duties and procedures.

Training should test and improve knowledge, provide simulations aimed at assessing attitudes, and unify the staff in its goals.

Family Issues 4

The primary focus of the early intervention program is the patient, but it is impossible to discuss early care without examining family dynamics. Alzheimer's disease is a cruel thief. It does not stop with robbing its victims of memory and, eventually, physical dignity. It also robs its victim's family and friends. Powerless to reverse the dementia, loved ones despair as the person they have known and loved gradually disappears until one day they see only an empty gaze from a familiar face.

This process takes 8 years on average and can last as long as 25. Despair need not be the automatic response to a diagnosis. Much can be done by and for caregivers and patients in the early stages. Support groups, home respite care, and day-care programs have proliferated for mid- to late-stage patients and caregivers. While commendable and necessary, this fails to raise family dynamics issues when most critical—at the onset. If these issues are addressed directly when the disease is first identified then the more demanding later stage care will not be as devastating for patient or caregiver.

Dr. Elisabeth Kübler-Ross's (1969) designation of the five stages of grief provides a framework for examining family issues in early stage care. The five stages are *denial, anger, bargaining, depression,* and *acceptance.* At least one stage will be present in each family's process. At any point the stages can overlap, and some stages will be absent entirely.

This chapter will examine the five stages and explore ways to cope with specific common problems.

DENIAL

One of the major barriers to early diagnosis is denial by both patient and caregiver. However, denial is not always intentional. Sometimes the denial is simply the result of ignorance. The patient or caregiver may attribute changes in behavior or lapses in memory to the normal process of aging. Early stage characteristics are not as dramatic and evident as mid- or late-life ones and can be readily confused with age-related problems. The major distinction is that Alzheimer's disease is progressive and disabling. Normal age-related memory loss is not.

A simple way to test the difference is to look closely at the patient's pattern of daily activities. Raise the issue of Alzheimer's disease and almost anyone will say, "I lose my keys all the time," or, "I always forget what I was going to do next." This is not Alzheimer's disease; it is short-term memory loss.

Eventually, usually in a short time, the keys will be found, the task remembered, and the job accomplished. By keeping written reminders, logging important events in a datebook, or using association to remember important names, the average aging person can carry on daily life.

The person with Alzheimer's disease doesn't just forget names. Whole sequences of words disappear. Basic tasks involving numbers, such as balancing checkbooks and paying bills, become impossible. The person may get lost when taking a familiar path home. Memory loss is significant and cannot be remedied with reminders such as datebooks or lists.

For such a person, incidents recur and grow more severe over time. To make matters worse, the patient sometimes forgets about forgetting. The patient literally doesn't remember failing to pay the bills and is surprised when the notices of intention to suspend services come in the mail.

In the beginning it is important for family and friends to listen carefully to conversations. An adult with normal memory loss might say, "The baby is crying. She must want her bottle now." For the moment, that adult cannot remember the baby's name, but can still recall that babies cry when hungry and wet. But an adult with dementia would be more likely to say, "That . . . she . . . you help her," and to point toward the screaming baby. Both the baby's name and the words for milk, bottle, and feeding would be lost, although the patient would struggle to appear to be aware of the problem and to suggest remedial action.

In the beginning the aphasia, or disruption of speech, is relatively mild. Familiar words do not come readily but speech is not totally impaired. Family and friends should listen closely for hesitation, circumlocution, and outright errors in speech use.

The early stage patient is a skilled dissembler, finding ways to disguise or excuse memory lapses, pointing out errors with a joke, or using other words when the right ones don't come readily to mind. All too often families and friends don't even notice the changes or lapses until a dramatic event—wandering in the streets until found by a stranger—brings attention to the situation. The changes are frightening for both patient and caregiver. Denial is one way to ease the fears.

In the movie *On Golden Pond,* the aging character played by Henry Fonda goes for a walk to collect berries for a pie. Walking a path he has taken for years he is suddenly overwhelmed by fear. He hears noises and sees movement. Momentarily confused, he cannot find the familiar way home. He runs, dropping the berries, and is finally relieved to stumble into the arms of his anxious wife. He quickly dismisses his fears, claiming that no berries are to be found and he is going back to his cabin. He lies about his terrors, denying the problem. This situation is magnified a hundredfold for the Alzheimer's patient, who truly does not know the way home but may be afraid that confession will mean loss of independence and admission of a terrifying future.

Fonda plays a gruff codger who rebuffs questions about his health with acerbic retorts. Rather than risk his ire, family and friends allow him to deny his increasing infirmities. Like Fonda's character, the Alzheimer's patient may minimize problems or try to dissuade questions by becoming thorny and intractable.

Too often, family and friends dismiss such personality changes as a sign of old age rather than a symptom of the onset of Alzheimer's disease. It is important to watch for distinct personality changes and to note if the changes are repeated and persistent.

Stereotypes of grumpy seniors often override the reality that irreversible personality changes have begun. If the patient is short-tempered when a mistake is discovered, it is often dismissed by others as the crankiness of aging. Outright cruelty and meanness are seen as a bitter response to aging rather than a sign of dementia and a signal that major personality changes are occurring. The patient is unlikely to admit that something is wrong or may, in fact, not even know the behavior is obvious to outsiders.

This is the time it is most important for friends and family to acknowledge the behavioral issues. As the disease progresses and the patient becomes increasingly less able to mask emotions, all the negative conflicts of the past will surface with increasing intensity. Petulance, manipulation, dependency—whatever the issues, they will intensify.

The patient will become increasingly less able to meet the caregivers' emotional needs. Demanding changes in behavior will not change the situation, because the patient *cannot* change. Understanding the behavior and developing an outside support network will help the caregiver or friend avoid inflammatory situations. It may be necessary for family members to enter therapy to deal with unresolved conflicts. Friends may need to learn to deal with loneliness, grief, or anger as the person they knew disappears.

Here the program director can play a useful role for the family. Directors should have a list of reliable support groups, therapists, and other professionals specializing in the issues. Directors should consider making it mandatory that relatives be in a support group before enrolling a patient in the program.

If there are problems in family dynamics it is likely these tensions will show outside the family circle. A patient may be cheerful during day care but grow silent or fearful when a spouse is near. A director should address such issues directly with family members. However, the director should be prepared for resistance or even anger from the family. The family usually comes to the program seeking solace and comradery, not questions about family dynamics or the suggestion that not all is well at home. Any intervention must be handled with great tact, otherwise the family may be embarrassed and withdraw the patient, or if there has been abuse may actually become more abusive.

It is not always possible for relatives to acknowledge the disease even after they have enrolled the patient in a program. In a few cases programs are oriented solely to activities, and discussion of the disease is deliberately precluded. These activities programs provide social outlets for patients and respite time for caregivers, which program planners may have deemed to be more important than confronting the long-term impact of the disease. On the whole, however, the sooner the family and patient confront the reality of the diagnosis, the sooner they can acquire as much information and help as possible.

Denial can also be a significant problem in practical matters such as finances. This is especially true if the affected partner is the one who managed the household affairs. Wills, property management, bank accounts, and other vital issues should be addressed while the patient still retains cognitive ability. Few will have made extensive preparations before the diagnosis, but there is time before the dementia progresses. Indeed, some professionals argue that it is an ethical mandate for the patient to have an active role in such matters (Brechling & Schneider, 1993).

Again, family members may be reluctant to deal with such matters, particularly wills and funeral plans. The advice of an attorney specializing in elder law will be beneficial at this point. Directors should keep a list of local attorneys.

The patient who lives alone poses a particular problem since changes in behavior can go unnoticed until there is a crisis such as a kitchen fire resulting from an unattended burner. It is important that relatives and friends learn about the patient's daily routines, perhaps by checking regularly with neighbors or visiting often enough to observe any warning signs.

Changes in behavior are not always the result of Alzheimer's disease. Stress, medication, alcohol or drug use, illness, or fatigue can all cause behavioral changes and exacerbate dementia. Elderly people who live alone are particularly susceptible to these conditions and often attempt to hide them.

Peg is a retired nurse. After her husband died she left the state and moved into a senior complex about a mile from her son Bob's home. She was close to shopping, movie theaters, and hiking trails. However, she missed her old friends and spent hours on the telephone. She told Bob that neighbors in the complex just didn't seem interested in being friends.

One day Bob got a call from one of Peg's old friends. Peg was now making her calls at 2 A.M. or later. She would talk incessantly about all the people she was helping at her new home, oblivious to her friends' sleepiness and the late hour.

When Bob confronted Peg she laughed and said she had probably just confused the time zones. She made Bob dinner and had several drinks during the evening. During dinner she told Bob about the people she had helped during the week. She said it was just like it used to be when she was a nurse.

As Bob left the apartment one of the neighbors stopped him. He angrily demanded to know why Bob's mother kept making 911 calls and disrupting the lives of her neighbors. The neighbor said Peg claimed to be a nurse who was trying to help out, but that she was calling ambulances and police officers for no reason. He wanted to have her evicted.

The next time Bob visited, Peg told him the same story and again she drank several drinks. Bob began to wonder if his mother might be drinking too much, but she was always well-groomed and seemed to be able to carry on with normal daily activities.

Bob talked with several friends about the situation, and one suggested that his mother might have some kind of dementia. He contacted the local Alzheimer's association and persuaded his mother to get diagnostic tests.

The doctor told Bob and Peg that she probably had Alzheimer's disease because she did not remember causing any trouble at the senior complex and did not think it was strange to call her friends at late hours. However, the doctor said other factors could be causing her strange behavior. Peg was very lonely and isolated. She was depressed and drinking heavily to avoid her feelings.

Bob moved Peg into a living center where she had her own quarters but ate communal meals and took part in an extensive social program.

In this case, at least two factors contributed to Peg's behavioral changes: stress and alcohol. Accustomed to his mother's social drinking and unwilling to face her loneliness, Bob denied the problems. The intervention of friends and neighbors forced Bob to confront the issues and to move Peg into a better situation.

These are the major facts to remember if denial is a factor in identifying early Alzheimer's disease.

- Age-related memory loss is not progressive or disabling. Alzheimer's disease is.
- Circumlocution, hesitation, and outright errors in speech use are signs of early aphasia.
- Marked behavioral changes usually signal dementia instead of the onset of old age.
- Ability to use numbers and to reason declines rapidly. The early stage is the time to put financial affairs in order. A lawyer can help.
- Factors such as poor nutrition, alcohol use, and stress contribute to dementia. People who live alone are especially subject to such factors.
- Caregivers should join a support group or consult a therapist before emotions get out of hand.

ANGER

Anger is perhaps the most frightening of responses to confront, and is almost universal for patients and caregivers. Anger is
almost always coupled with other emotions, most often guilt,
shame, fear, and grief.

When talking about the patient, caregivers sometimes say that
before the disease was diagnosed they thought the patient was
being annoying on purpose.

> Jane, 72, was married to Bob, 75, for 10 years. The couple met at
> church, married within a few months, and immediately left on a
> church mission to Africa. Bob, a retired engineer, was put in
> charge of a water project, and Jane, a retired teacher, gave health
> education classes. Within the first month in Africa Bob began
> having problems. He was supposed to supervise a crew installing a
> pipeline, a job he had done hundreds of times. He kept making
> mistakes and blaming the crew.
>
> Bob would not talk to Jane, although she begged him, cried, and
> eventually even screamed at him. He responded to her outbursts
> with silence and despair. One day Bob exploded at the crew, angry
> that they had laid the wrong size pipe in a trench, pipe that Bob
> himself had ordered. The mission director heard about the incident
> and sent Jane and Bob back home.
>
> Jane thought Bob would be comfortable back in their own apart-
> ment, but she began to notice other problems. He couldn't balance
> the checkbook, he didn't return important calls, and he sometimes
> forgot her name. She persuaded Bob to see his family physician,
> who did extensive tests and told them that Bob probably had
> Alzheimer's disease.

Jane's anger was replaced with shame. When the problems
started in Africa, she had thought Bob was being stubborn, too
proud to admit that life in a foreign country was harder than he
had thought it would be. She had never suspected that he could
not remember how to measure pipe. She had been scared that he
might want a divorce if she continued to confront him, so she had
let the behavior continue until the mission director intervened.

Now she realizes that Bob had serious memory losses and needed help.

When people do not understand why a relationship is changing they typically respond with anger. If the patient handles the family's business dealings, the spouse will become angry when the patient makes mistakes in the checkbook and bill payments and endangers their financial security. The patient may then grow angry in turn, insisting on carrying on even though incapable. If the patient leaves the door unlocked despite repeated nagging, the spouse's nagging will grow worse. Or the patient and spouse may withdraw into silence and cut each other off, as Bob and Jane did in Africa. Anger will soon divide even the closest of families.

Friends may feel neglected and get angry because the patient becomes unreliable, missing dinner dates or failing to return calls. Sometimes the patient's behavior changes just enough to reawaken old conflicts, giving a sour edge to casual conversations and interactions. The friendship may not seem worth saving. This is anger at the first level, anger at changes that are not understood and may even appear deliberate. This is the time to look closely at the behavior, to question whether the relationship has major problems or whether the spouse or friend is exhibiting behavior typical of dementia.

But anger often does not disappear when the diagnosis is confirmed. In fact, it usually intensifies. Like Jane, a spouse may be ashamed of having missed the warning signals. Or a dependent spouse or friend may become even more angry upon realizing that total loss is impending.

The spouse or friend may accuse the patient of abandonment even while knowing the blame is irrational. Or, the spouse or friend may turn the full force of the anger onto the patient, exploding at shortcomings, and refusing to accept things the patient can no longer control. This kind of anger can harm both the patient and others, since the demands can never be met. This kind of anger is not directed solely to the patient. Spouse or friends may become angry at other people, systems, and even God. The doctor should have done something sooner, insurance companies should cover the bills but don't, and God acts un-reasonably and allows good people to get hurt, become sick, and die.

The common factor in each rage is a sense of helplessness. It is far easier to turn the rage on anything rather than accept the progressive loss and loneliness. Yet it is not appropriate to sup-press anger. It does not work to repress anger. If it is stuffed down it will only intensify, exploding in disproportionate form just as the patient deteriorates further and needs more attention.

It is important and appropriate for patient and caregiver to acknowledge the anger—the patient, anger at loss of capacity; the caregiver, anger at loss of companion. It is appropriate and even necessary for patient and caregiver to confront God, to question the senselessness and cruelty of what is happening.

But it is necessary to be realistic about this anger. Anger will not stop the disease's progression. Anger at the patient will not improve the situation, and will, in fact, increase stress and lower the patient's coping mechanisms. Anger will not produce a cure for the disease, provide insurance coverage, or pay bills. Anger may even slow the system. The clerk who has been the target of anger may delay paperwork as a payback, or fail to bring a letter to the attention of a supervisor.

Finding an outlet for this level of anger is vital. Solace may be more welcome than rage at this point, but it is rage that is necessary. A minister may say that suffering is God's will, but this ignores the emotional pain of the one who comes for advice. Sacred scriptures of all faiths encourage believers to be honest with God about emotions. Indeed, in sacred scriptures, God is often depicted as angry, impatient, and full of questions about why life is as it is. To suggest that to have faith means to accept suffering is to belie the healing power of anger. If the family is unable to do so for themselves, the director should help them find a minister or counselor who will encourage full release of feelings.

A good first step for releasing anger is to acknowledge it in writing. Simply putting the words "I am angry" in print makes the feeling seem more valid. Then the angry person can expand the statement to include the specific things triggering the anger:

fear of financial loss, sorrow over loss of companionship, helplessness to change bureaucratic structures.

It is also important to remember that anger will recur throughout the stages of the disease. The goal is not to eliminate anger but to understand and control it.

These are key ways to manage anger:

- Anger is always mixed with other emotions such as guilt, shame, fear, or grief. Expect these feelings to surface.
- If a relationship is troubling, examine it and determine whether it is flawed or whether dementia is beginning.
- Acknowledge and vent anger with professional guidance. Do not use crutches such as "this must be God's will" to repress anger.
- Do not misdirect anger. It can harm the patient directly and indirectly.

BARGAINING

Bargaining is generally the briefest stage in the process. Bargaining is a way to try to delay the inevitable. The patient or caregiver strikes a short-lived bargain which quickly gives way to the realities of the disease.

The patient or family may know of the problem but decide to attempt daily normal activity as long as possible. "Well, I'll only drive the car to the market. I won't go on long trips any more." Then the day comes when the patient forgets he drove to the market and walks home. Or, "The apartment is small. I can manage for a while." Then the patient leaves the oven burners on all day. No damage is done but the chances of starting a fire the next time are high.

Some bargaining may be useful if it allows the patient to remain dignified and continue daily routines. However, when the bargain is unrealistic and results in danger to the patient and others, it should be ended quickly and no other bargain struck.

Patient and caregiver may also try to bargain with God, usually in the form of prayers. The belief that prayer will be heard is comforting in even the worst situations. Prayers for the courage to cope with the disease or discernment of the best ways to live out the remaining days are realistic pleas. However, it is important to remember that a prayer for a cure is little more than wishful thinking and is unlikely to be answered.

Everyone bargains. Sometimes it is useful and comforting.

- Useful bargains enable the patient to continue daily routines or enhance the patient's dignity.
- Prayer is a form of bargaining with God and can provide comfort, but it should not be an unrealistic demand.
- If bargaining results in danger to self or others the bargain should be ended.

DEPRESSION

Like anger, depression is a significant and recurring state in the entire process of the disease. It is common in both patients' and caregivers' lives.

The advent of such medications as Prozac has focused public attention on depression and raised public awareness of how to recognize depression. Put simply, depression is a long-term state of feeling blue. Among its symptoms are change in eating patterns, weight loss or gain, inability to sleep, fatigue, inability to concentrate, and the constant sense that life is meaningless. Other signs are short temper, a tendency to cry, unusual forgetfulness, and a tendency to withdraw from social contacts.

Caregivers generally have a clear cause for their depression. They must deal with the stress of planning for future care, knowledge of pending loss, and even changes in the attitudes of well-meaning friends and family. Although caregivers may in fact be able to carry on lives nearly normally during the early stage, even the knowledge of what is going to happen will be sufficient enough to trigger depression for some caregivers.

Depression is a normal and natural part of the grieving process. As with anger, it will do no good to repress the emotions. Having a support group or counselor is critical at this stage. It is completely normal to feel sad about the loss and fearful about the work ahead, but it may be difficult for caregivers to admit they are grieving.

Because of the widespread publicity about antidepressants, some caregivers may be tempted to seek medication. If at all possible this should be avoided. Use of antidepressants, though likely to make the situation seem more bearable, may, in fact, interfere with the normal grieving process. If, however, depression persists and deepens to the point that it interferes with daily activities, then the caregiver should see a doctor for advice. If a doctor prescribes antidepressants the caregiver should still join a support group or see a counselor on a regular basis. Peer support is critical in the grieving process.

Recognizing the reasons for the patient's depression can be more difficult. The patient will be affected by many of the same factors as the caregiver, including fear of the future and changes in the attitudes of loved ones. But among other factors that could be triggering depression for the patient are insufficient sunlight, prescription drugs, thyroid disease, diabetes, poor nutrition, or lack of exercise ("10 Physical Reasons," 1992).

Here the day-care program becomes a critical factor in reducing or eliminating many of the causes of depression.

A critical component of the successful day-care program is exercise (Lindemuth & Moose, 1990). Even simple activities such as basic gymnastics, short walks, or throwing a ball back and forth provides necessary stimuli.

The program intake process should be thorough and include full discussion of the patient's medical history, eating habits, and prescription history. This will enable the program director to identify reasons why a patient might be depressed. Even when the evaluation is thorough, some things may escape notice.

Jan is a 67-year-old woman enrolled in the Weeks Day Care Center. On alternate weeks the patients brought bag lunches to the center.

The first week Jan brought two beers and an orange. The director took the beers and shared her sandwich with Jan. Two weeks later Jan again brought beer. Again the director took the beer, this time giving Jan her entire lunch because Jan appeared to be ravenous. The third time this happened the director gave Jan no food. She called Jan's family to discuss the problem.

Jan's daughter was surprised but not disturbed. She said her mother always had a beer with her meals and had not had any problems with alcoholism. However, she believed Jan when Jan told her the refrigerator was fully stocked. When she checked her mother's apartment she found that Jan had beer, fruit, bread, and little else.

Thereafter the daughter went shopping with Jan and made certain she prepared and ate balanced meals. As an extra precaution she had a community agency deliver Jan a hot meal on weekdays.

Jan was happier and took part in the activities more readily after she started eating regular nutritious meals. Both her family and the director learned to monitor her food intake and to question her about what she had eaten when she appeared to be depressed.

One telltale sign of depression in Alzheimer's patients is a change in self-care. A previously immaculately groomed patient may become unkempt, slovenly, or simply dirty. A man may have stubble or a woman may have greasy hair. Either may fail to button clothing, or wear the same soiled sweater week after week.

Abrupt changes in appearance usually indicate that the patient has given up hope. It is important to encourage early stage patients to groom themselves, dress nicely, and present themselves in a socially acceptable manner. As the disease progresses they will be incapable of personal care and the caregiver will have to groom the patient, but in the beginning the patient is capable of self-care and should not be allowed to neglect personal care.

This is what to remember about depression:

- Caregivers may become depressed in the early stages because they are worried about what is going to happen in the future.
- A depressed caregiver should only take antidepressants if the depression interferes with daily activities.
- Antidepressants should only be taken after a consultation with a doctor, and in conjunction with therapy and group support.
- Lack of light, poor nutrition, and many other factors can trigger depression.
- Decline in self-care in the early stages signals depression.

ACCEPTANCE

Not every family or patient will accept a diagnosis and some will refuse to discuss the disease at all. For these people, the term of the disease is apt to be filled with emotional problems, financial concerns, and increasing social isolation.

For those who attempt to accept the diagnosis and deal with the implications, the early stage is a time for planning and can be a time of relative peace.

This is the time when the family and patient can and should make necessary legal preparations. The patient can help draft a will and a durable power of attorney for health care (see Appendix D), including specific remarks about being a research subject. This is the time when the patient should dispose of possessions. It is also a time to clear up emotional issues with family members and friends, with the caveat that family and friends should understand the limits of the patient's abilities to reason and be logical. It is an ideal time for the patient to prepare a legacy such as scrapbook or memoirs.

Caregivers can guide this process with the aid of attorneys and other trusted professionals. The tasks should be undertaken at the times in the day when the patient is in top mental and physical condition. The tasks should be spaced out over time rather than undertaken in one surge that becomes an intense emotional pressure.

Planning for health care cannot be deferred. Private Alzheimer's facilities are expensive. Special units in nursing homes accept Medicaid patients but the waiting lists are long. It is unrealistic to expect to find a bed suddenly just because it is wanted or needed. Many nursing homes will not accept Alzheimer's patients at any price, so the patient may have to be placed some distance from home.

Once plans are made, payment arrangements must be clear. Private-pay facilities charge an average of $3,000 per month and will soon deplete most patients' savings. Public aid will not be available if the patient still has savings even if these savings are administered by a conservator. Few families are realistic about the enormous financial burden of Alzheimer's care. The patient can linger on for years, exhausting even the wealthiest family's resources.

Families that have no serious financial worries still cope with the guilt of placing a relative in long-term care. The process will be easier for all if the patient has a say in what is going to happen. The process can bring peace to a family. Knowing, rather than guessing, what a patient wants enables the caregiver to do what is necessary at each stage without excessive guilt or shame. Planning ahead enables the caregiver to get optimal treatment at affordable rates. Finally, helping the patient to put affairs in order and constructing memoirs can actually bring families closer together.

Directors can help in this process by keeping a list of elder law attorneys and social workers specializing in gerontology. Each county has an ombudsman, an agent designated by the federal government to watch over the welfare of people in institutions. The ombudsman will have a list of licensed Alzheimer's facilities and information about admission standards. The ombudsman may also help choose an appropriate facility and smooth the way for admission.

Many issues can be resolved in early stage.

- Financial and health-care decisions should be made while the patient is still able to take part.
- The program director, an elder law attorney, a geriatric social worker, or the county ombudsman can help facilitate planning.

BEYOND THE FIVE STAGES: THE EARLY INTERVENTION GROUP

Support groups can be a place where patients can talk with others about common experiences. However, the decision for a patient to enter a support group should be made by patient and family together. If a patient doesn't want to come then the group won't do the patient any good. A group should not become a dumping ground for beleaguered families.

Patient, family, and group leader should agree from the onset how much is to be shared outside the group. In most cases it is vital for directors to discuss behavior issues, health problems, and similar issues with family members. However, it is not necessary to convey all the personal emotions and private thoughts to family members. Patients need a safe place to vent anger, fears, and other emotions without worry that their privacy will be violated. Families should be encouraged to leave the site and not to use the program as *their* emotional support.

Consider the case of John, 45, whose wife developed severe aphasia at age 43. John always brought Ruth to the weekly meeting. In the first few weeks he would joke with staff and patients who arrived early, delaying the start of the program by up to 15 minutes.

As time went on he tended to stay longer and to break down, often crying and saying how hard it was to see Ruth so affected. Then he began to do the same thing when he came to pick up Ruth. John's problems demanded at least an hour of staff time each week, and Ruth was often agitated by his crying and the staff's obvious discomfort.

Finally the director spoke to John and asked him to meet her at the door to deliver and pick up Ruth. She urged John to join a support group but John would not. Instead he began calling the director at home, engaging her in long conversations about his problems.

John's demands were overwhelming and the director needed to insist that he get outside help. A director should be equally wary of families that have no contact with the program. There may be valid reasons why the family is unable to bring the patient to the center. However, all families should complete an initial interview with the director, and periodic meetings, at least monthly, should be scheduled at mutually agreeable times.

At this point existing early care programs charge low fees, making programs readily accessible to anyone interested. Nevertheless, payment arrangements should be clear at time of enrollment, including the issue of payment for missed sessions.

As programs become more sophisticated, or if they become part of a medical plan, fees may rise. In that case it is imperative that fees be handled prior to enrollment. In no case should a patient be enrolled in a program if it is clear that the family cannot afford it. It is cruel and counterproductive to take the patient away from new friends and activities.

These are preliminary things to consider when looking for an early stage program.

- The support group is not the place for the family to work out its issues.
- Families must have sustained contact with the director but should not be allowed to use the director as a substitute therapist.
- The patient's privacy is the foremost concern of the support group. Family members can be told essential information but the patient's emotional revelations should be treated with respect.

• Early stage care is affordable but financial arrangements should be clearly stated and payments received regularly.

CONCLUSION

Many issues arise for families during the early stage. Among these are anger, guilt, and financial fears. The early stage is the time when families and patients can most benefit from a realistic look at the disease and its impact, but is the time when people are most likely to deny, bargain, or otherwise evade necessary emotional and financial tasks.

Families cope best when given information about early stage issues. It is important to know what triggers or masks depression and behavior changes.

It is necessary to learn about financial and health-care options while the patient can take part in the process.

Facing the issues can bring peace and long-term financial security to both patients and families.

Screening
Participants

5

The identification and selection of participants for an early intervention program should be a careful process. Existing groups are small and require intense personal interactions. Choice of members who are unable to take part fully in the activities will seriously affect the entire program.

The board should decide whether the program will be for men, women, or both sexes. Race, socioeconomic status, and religion should not be barriers to admission. To the contrary, efforts should be made to diversify the membership. Physical disability should not be a bar unless the candidate is incapable of doing the activities.

Both patient and caregivers should take part in the selection process. It is vital for the screening committee to have both perspectives on the patient's condition. The family should never speak for the patient.

The early intervention program is primarily for the patient, although a few programs have concomitant family support groups. The family must understand that the structure and goals of the program are not designed to deal with family dynamic issues except in tangental fashion. It is appropriate for families to seek a separate support group for counseling.

In some cases the patient will have neither family nor caregiver, but will have undergone a battery of tests and been given a diagnosis. In that case it is appropriate to screen the patient for admission, but with the caveat that critical interaction with outside observers will not happen. The staff will have to bear a greater burden in assessing the patient's progress in the program and have less likelihood of finding out what outside factors contribute to a decline in capacity.

The screening committee must establish criteria for admission. Each candidate should have a medical diagnosis prior to application. Other criteria can include: high scores on the Mini-Mental Exam, continence, control of undesirable or dangerous behaviors, and any other appropriate selectors.

Screening is the time when policies are explained, including attendance requirements, financial arrangements, and termination procedures. It is also the time when transportation of the patient, particular medical needs, and liability are established.

Finally, the screening gives the patient a chance to voice some preliminary concerns. These include being stigmatized for having the disease, lessening or giving up driving, becoming more dependent on other people, and preparing for the future.

PRELIMINARY SCREENING

A patient who is incontinent, or wanders, or has severe behavioral problems should never be considered for an early care program. The patient could well achieve a high score on standard mental exams and might really want to be a group member, but in a short time would become a burden and undermine the program.

Staff members of early intervention groups are not qualified to diagnose Alzheimer's disease. Granada Hills Community Hospital in Granada, California, requires that all candidates have interviews with a psychologist and a speech therapist, but even these professionals are not qualified to do the necessary medical evaluation.

Only patients who have been diagnosed by a physician should be considered for a program. Not only will the doctor have done the necessary medical and neurological confirmation of the disease's presence, but the doctor will also be available to monitor the patient's progressive dementia and to deal with any medical problems or emergencies.

Some early stage groups are little more than social clubs. A family that is denying or avoiding the diagnosis may try to use membership as a way to show that nothing serious is wrong with the patient. Even if the primary goal of the club is social activity the director should insist upon a medical diagnosis and the family's acknowledgement of the diagnosis.

A thorough examination for dementia includes a mental status exam, usually the Mini-Mental State Exam. Most early care groups require a score of at least 15 on this test for admission. However, the Early Birds Support Group of Honolulu, Hawaii, notes that the exam only tests functional ability, not the patient's ability to discuss feelings ("Early Birds Support Group Summary," 1991). Therefore high scores should not be the only criteria for admission, particularly if the group intends to have regular discussions of issues.

Under no circumstances should a director accept a patient because of pressure from a family. Caregivers may be desperate for respite, unwilling to acknowledge the patient's limitations, or not concerned about what the patient wants.

These are preliminary screening criteria:

- Patients with uncontrollable behaviors, incontinence, or who wander should not be admitted.
- All group members must have a medical diagnosis prior to admission.
- High mental test scores are not sufficient criteria for admission.
- Resist pressure from family members.

SCREENING THE FAMILY

The involvement of family or caregivers in a patient's care plan can make a difference in the patient's progress—for good or bad.

Screening by Telephone

Most of the detrimental effects of family involvement have already been discussed. The family may actively deny any problems, cover up for the patient, avoid dealing with unpleasant or dangerous behavior until there is a crisis, or simply be ignorant of the gravity of the situation.

Any such attitudes must be uncovered in the first round of discussion, which can readily be done by telephone. The family should be able to say how the dementia first came to someone's attention and who then made the medical diagnosis.

Then the family should discuss feelings about the diagnosis, the patient's care, and impact on family life. This is the time to determine how the family is coping with its own issues and whether the family has sought support from a counselor or a group.

If the family appears to have acknowledged the diagnosis and is coping with changes, then it is appropriate to ask about the patient. The family should be able to report any behavior problems, medical difficulties, or other impairments that might preclude participation. These matters will be discussed more thoroughly later by both family and patient, so brief answers are sufficient.

The family should say whether it seems likely the patient can cope with a social setting for at least two hours. If the patient has other problems such as physical disabilities this is the time to say so.

The family should also state whether the decision to come to the program is mutual. If it is not, then the family should say whether or not the patient has been told the diagnosis and why. If the patient has not been told, the family should explain what the patient thinks the program is designed to do.

Although it is not mandatory that every patient know about the diagnosis it is preferable. No patient should be accepted if it is obvious the family is trying to hide the truth from the patient because the probability is high that the patient will hear the truth from other group members.

The family should discuss whether members can handle the requirements of participation such as arranging for transportation to and from the site, paying fees, and meeting regularly with the director.

The family should also state expectations of the program, particularly the length of time they expect the patient to be a group member. The family should show awareness that the disease is progressive and group membership will be temporary.

If the screening committee is satisfied with the answers to all these questions, then the caller should confirm the patient's interest in the group by speaking directly to the patient. If the family will not allow the patient to answer questions, the candidate should not be admitted.

If the patient indicates interest in the program, then it is appropriate to set up a meeting time with the patient and family. At that meeting the director or screening committee will speak with the patient and family, together and separately.

It is possible to do a preliminary screening by telephone.

- The family should be aware of the medical diagnosis and be able to discuss it.
- The family should have feelings about the diagnosis and life-style changes and should be getting help from a support group or counselor.
- The decision should be mutual and the family should agree to let the patient confirm that by telephone.
- The family should be able to handle entrance requirements such as fees and transportation.
- The family should acknowledge that the program can only be temporary.

The First Meeting

It is important for the director and other screening committee members to see firsthand how a family interacts. Therefore it is appropriate to conduct at least part of the interview process with both family and patients together.

The questions asked when the family and patient are together should be brief and general. The major goal of the joint meeting is not to get verbal information but to observe family dynamics. If the director asks vital questions when family and patient are together, such as an assessment of mental health, the family may exaggerate the patient's abilities and the patient may follow that lead. If such vital questions are asked separately and compared a more accurate portrait will emerge.

The director should note whether family members allow a patient to answer questions without prompting. The family should be encouraged to supplement the patient's answers but if the patient is being ignored then it is likely that the patient also had little role in the decision to come to the center. The patient, not the family, should be the one to describe the patient's hobbies and interests.

Sometimes a family will speak as though the patient were not even in the room, or speak of the patient only in the third person. This depersonalizing way of talking about an intimate companion indicates that the family has already distanced themselves from any painful feelings likely to occur because of the patient. This is a subtle clue that the family will not provide enough home support for a patient and the patient is probably not a good candidate for the program.

The director can determine whether the family actually sees and responds to problem behaviors, or glosses over them with pity, condescension, or irritation. It is also important to be aware of how much the family has to help the patient with routine acts such as sitting or how they respond to speech and hearing deficits. If the family has already developed dependent patterns, the patient will probably expect the same in a program and will not be prepared to cope when asked to be independent.

It is possible to assess family dynamics by watching the interaction of patient and family. The director should note whether the patient is tense or relaxed, fearful or confident, and quiet or talkative. In this case, body language may also say what words do not. Do family members touch the patient frequently or not at all, rebuff or ignore any advances by the patient, or take a domineering posture over the patient?

A certain amount of restraint should be expected since this is a strange situation, but the deeper dynamics are still likely to be evident. When the director has thoroughly observed personal interactions then separate interviews can be held with family and patient. If the patient tires easily during the joint interview it may be appropriate to schedule the separate interview for another day.

The separate family interview will be a thorough discussion of how the family perceives the patient's abilities. This will include many questions about how the patient copes with daily living, overall mood assessment, any particular behavioral problems, whether the patient's routines have changed, and how the patient spends an average day.

The family will also discuss how they are involved with the patient and whether that has changed. They will explain how they feel about discussing the disease with the patient. They will also explain whether other people know about the diagnosis and how the family feels about that.

This interview has at least two purposes: First, the director will compare the patient's self-perception with the family's and try to gauge the patient's mental status; second, the director will learn whether the family or patient feel any stigma about the disease.

The first meeting has several vital functions.

- The joint interview is the best way to observe family dynamics and determine whether the family really knows the impact of dementia.

- The family can provide vital information about the patient's mental status and give the director something to compare against the patient's self-perception.
- The director can note disturbing family problems or stigma.

Subsequent Meetings

If the family appears to meet the criteria then at least one meeting should be scheduled prior to the start of the program to handle business matters.

Any decisions reached at that meeting should be put in writing so that no misunderstandings will occur later. The family should specify who will transport the patient to and from meetings.

All fees should be paid in advance or arrangement made for payment at each session. High functioning patients can be included in payment plans but in general trying to handle money is a major issue for early care patients. If possible the patient should not be given the responsibility of carrying cash, as it can be lost or stolen.

The family should give the director a list of important contacts such as the doctor and other family members, including at least two people who can assume responsibility for the patient if the family is unavailable. If required, the family member should sign a release for emergency medical treatment. As needed the family should sign consent forms or release of liability for field trips.

The family should note in writing any special medical problems including allergies, food intolerance, or physical disabilities. The form should include a list of any medications and dosages, whether the patient will bring the medicine, and when the patient should take the dose. The family should understand that any medicine should be locked up when the patient arrives so that someone else does not accidentally take it.

The family should also agree not to allow the patient to bring valuables or sentimental keepsakes to the program site. The risk of theft, damage, or of forgetting to take the objects home is high.

Finally, the family should understand how much of the

patient's progress will be private and how much will be shared, and agree to honor those boundaries.

This is an appropriate time for the director to give the family lists of resources, particularly if the program does not have a family support component.

Subsequent meetings can be scheduled by family or director and can include the exchange of information about support programs and counseling about specific problems. Such sessions are primarily for the family's benefit. In addition, the director should schedule regular meetings with the family to discuss the patient's progress and the impact on family dynamics. Any medical or behavioral issues should be reported and resolved.

Each family will meet with the director several times.

- Just prior to the beginning of the program the family will meet with the director to complete business matters.
- The family and director can choose to meet periodically to discuss the family's personal issues.
- The family and director should hold regular meetings to discuss the patient's medical and behavioral problems and progress in the program.

SCREENING THE PATIENT

The patient must be a willing participant in the program. It is appropriate to involve the patient in the selection process as soon as it evident that no physical or behavioral problems are a bar to admission. The most reliable evidence is the medical exam.

Screening by Telephone

As indicated, the first contact can be by telephone. This should be brief; it is sufficient to ask whether the patient wants to attend the group and is willing to be interviewed. Keeping in mind that the patient may have mild aphasia or be confused, ask the two questions separately and slowly.

Avoid getting into long discussions by telephone because the early stage patient is easily confused and has many fears. The patient may mistakenly believe that a family member has already made the decision, or fear that he or she is being taken to a nursing home.

The First Meeting

In addition to noting interaction with family, the director will have a separate interview with the patient. This interview has many functions: 1) to compare the patient's self-assessment against the family's; 2) to conduct a brief mental test; 3) to learn more about the patient's feelings about the diagnosis; and 4) to discuss the program.

The director should ask the patient the same questions the family answered. These include detailed questions about memory loss, unusual behavior, daily living habits, social activities, interaction with family members, and moods and emotions.

These questions should be asked one at a time and slowly. The director should allow the patient a lot of time to answer and should not attempt to suggest words. The answers should reflect as accurately as possible the patient's own terminology and limitations. If the patient cannot answer something or is too embarrassed the director should go on to the next question.

The director will be looking for obvious discrepancies between the patient's account and the family's. If the two accounts nearly coincide then the patient is a likely candidate for the program. If the patient perceives no problem and is unaware of behavior, then the patient probably does not have enough grasp on reality to succeed in a program.

The director will ask the patient whether the patient has experienced any major changes. If the patient admits to memory loss or one of the other early-stage behaviors, then the director should ask what the patient thinks the problem is. If the patient says it is Alzheimer's disease the director should ask how the patient knows this. It is not uncommon for a patient to know the truth even though the family believes the patient knows nothing about having the disease. In that case the real problem is the avoidance behavior of the family.

If the patient seems inclined to do so, this is the time to talk about any emotional responses to the diagnosis. The patient may feel like a burden to the family, want to die now, be frightened, or still wonder if the doctor made a mistake.

The director should find out what the patient thinks is likely to happen in the future. The director should determine whether the patient has sought other help, perhaps counseling by a geriatrics social worker or a psychiatrist, drug treatments, or other support groups.

The director should ask why the patient wants to enroll in the early stage group. The patient should describe what he or she believes will happen in the group. This is the time to find out whether the patient likes to be in groups, has been in other groups recently, and wants sustained social interaction.

This is also the time the director will learn what the patient's interests and skills are. The director should encourage the patient to talk about hobbies, attendance at church or synagogue, travel, professional affiliations, and whatever else the patient does on a regular basis.

Asking questions about expectations, previous group experience, and interests will help the director determine whether the patient will really enjoy the program and benefit from being in it. Someone who has never been in a group or dislikes discussions is not a good candidate. Nor is anyone who dislikes singing, crafts, and other activities that are routine parts of most groups.

The director will test the patient's mental status. The Mini-Mental State Exam is short, easy, and non-threatening. It may even be familiar to the patient who has already been tested. The director should explain that it is just a tool to test memory, not a test of whether the patient is good or bad. The patient who cannot answer the test questions is unlikely to be able to follow simple directions and is a poor candidate for the program.

This may also be the time the patient talks about issues such as not being able to drive, or losing friends, but it is equally appropriate to discuss such issues at another session just before the program begins. The director should gauge how tired the patient is before including those issues in the first interview.

The director can learn many things about a patient during the interview.

- The patient's self-assessment may be radically different than the family's.
- The patient may know about the diagnosis and understand what it means.
- The patient's personal experiences and interests may make it likely that the patient would neither enjoy nor benefit from the group.

Subsequent Meetings

If the patient seems a likely candidate for the group, the director might schedule several other meetings before the program begins. This will offer the director a chance to observe the patient's long-term behavior, note the patient's concerns, and allow the patient to become comfortable with the director.

The director may choose to discuss some of the more predominant concerns with the patient before the program begins. The patients will then discuss the concerns among themselves when the program begins. They are generally pleased to learn that other people have had the same problems, and may find new solutions or ways to accept what they did.

Many early stage patients still drive but are concerned about it. These drivers tend to stay close to home, drive only when necessary, and avoid carrying passengers. Even the prudent driver usually has fears about having an accident and being forced to give up the license, thereby losing independence. The patient knows that the time will come when the law will require giving up the license but hopes to stall that day as long as possible.

Dependency is a constant issue. Many patients are trying to cope with diminished skills that have changed their role in the family. This is especially true if the patient still worked or was managing the family finances. Now the patient must depend entirely on someone else to handle essential tasks.

The patient is extremely sensitive to changing family dynamics. Most patients talk openly about not wanting to be a burden to the family but are afraid of being placed in a nursing home. Most want desperately to control the dementia but realize that it is impossible. They hope that their families will not become too angry or upset with them, but can already sense impatience when they make mistakes.

Friends seem to draw away or become unreliable just when the patient needs them most. Sometimes friends are frightened by the changes and perhaps even fearful of also getting the disease. Other friends may not be able to face the progressive loss and just abruptly end the relationship. Some friends try to comfort the patient by voicing false optimism about the future, when what the patient wants is for someone to understand how bad it really is.

The patient faces incredible stigma. As has been discussed extensively, few people know much about the disease and are unaware that the early stage patient can carry on a near-normal life for years. People may believe the disease is contagious, a result of something bad the patient did, or a declaration that the patient is already completely crazy. People stop talking to the patient, or talk down to the patient. The patient soon feels like an object and not a person.

The patient is concerned about the future. This is not limited to fears of being placed in a nursing home or knowledge that the disease is terminal. The patient may have very clear ideas about wills, funerals, health care directives, and other legal matters, but may find that family members consider the patient too demented to make any decisions.

The patient is almost always interested in research and often willing to be the subject for an experimental drug or procedure. Again, the family may not allow the patient to agree to research, perhaps fearful that the drug will actually shorten the time left or increase the dementia. Or the patient or family may have false hopes about the experimental procedure.

Finally, the patient may be frustrated at not being able to communicate clearly. It is common to see an early stage patient struggle to find a word, turn red, and break into tears or become angry when language fails. The patient knows very well what is wrong but cannot find the words to say it.

A NOTE ON PATIENTS WITH NO FAMILY OR CAREGIVER

The solo patient is a particular concern because so much of his or her life is hidden. No one knows if the patient eats balanced meals, stays up all night crying, or drinks too much.

The director should stay in close contact with the solo patient's physician and report any problems to the doctor. The doctor is bound by an oath of confidentiality and cannot talk to the director about the patient's file, but can take note of the director's concerns and talk to the patient if necessary.

The director should also visit the solo patient occasionally to see if everything is going smoothly. That is the best place to chat with neighbors who might notice if the patient has behaved strangely, been ill, or been absent for a prolonged time.

It is also appropriate for the director to find out who the people are the patient sees regularly and get to know them. A close friend or the neighborhood grocery clerk might provide valuable information when it is needed.

The solo patient is often very independent and will react unfavorably to the suggestion of moving in with someone else and giving up personal space. If this appears to be necessary the director could suggest the patient consider a retirement center with private living quarters but shared meals and activities.

CONCLUSION

Identification of ideal candidates for an early stage program requires careful screening of both family and patient. The family may not know what the patient wants or needs, or may have selfish motives for putting the patient in a program. On the other hand, the family may know more about the patient's limits and problems than the patient does. The patient may not be interested in a program or may not have the behavioral or physical skills to do the activities. Or the patient may be overwhelmed with concerns that could be fruitfully addressed in a program.

Decisions will have to be made one at a time since there are no criteria for automatic selection. This means that the process will be demanding and time-consuming. On the other hand, the chosen candidates are unlikely to have hidden problems or agendas and are more likely to benefit from the program.

Identifying and Coping with Common Behaviors

6

Patients in the early stages of dementia do not exhibit many of the problem behaviors that often emerge as the disease progresses. Such problem behaviors include hitting, screaming, crying, resisting assistance, intense and prolonged agitation, preoccupation with leaving the site, incontinence, and paranoia.

However, early stage patients do exhibit behaviors that can be a problem if the staff is not prepared to recognize and cope with them. Among such behaviors are confusion, an urgent need to toilet, anger, failure to remember words, unpredictable or inappropriate responses, momentary agitation, stubbornness, and venting emotions greater than the situation seems to merit.

Before taking any action in a situation, it is important for staff to determine the cause of the behavior. Possibilities are:

1. The staff may be causing the behavior, either intentionally or inadvertently.
2. Other patients may be causing the problem.
3. The patient may have other problems, such as an adverse reaction to medication, an illness, or a problem at home.

85

4. The client may simply be exhibiting behaviors characteristic of the dementia.

When the cause of the behavior has been established the staff should deal promptly with the situation. Comprehensive staff training includes role plays of situations involving these behaviors and extensive discussion of ways to resolve the problems. (See Chapter 3.) The well-trained staff should not be surprised if these behaviors arise and should be able to deal with them with minimum disruption to the daily program.

RECOGNIZING PROBLEM BEHAVIORS

The screening process should eliminate patients whose behaviors make them unsuitable for an early care program. However, occasionally someone will enroll who appears to be high functioning but whose behavior becomes borderline or unsuitable during the actual program.

> Sam was continent, alert, able to communicate readily, and capable of doing the program's activities.
>
> However, when introduced to the group, Sam took a complete dislike to another patient, Joe. He avoided Joe as much as possible, but the whole group ate lunch at one table. During lunch Joe accidentally dropped his fork near Sam's seat, and tried to apologize, but Sam began shouting at Joe. The outburst was brief, but Sam continued to glare at Joe for the rest of the day. Joe avoided coming near Sam for the rest of the day. The rest of the group also looked nervously at Sam and two men avoided sitting near him.
>
> This situation, unfortunately, had no resolution. The director talked to Sam and found out that Joe reminded him of his estranged son. Sam was completely overcome with emotion as he talked about his son. "That Joe reminds me so much of him," Sam told the director. "I just look at Joe and I get mad about what Bill did."
>
> Sam knew that Joe was not his son, but had been unable to

control his anger because Joe reminded him so much of his son Bill. Sam's dementia had affected his ability to control his emotions.

The director gave Sam another chance, but the next week, Sam avoided Joe and glared across the room at him. It was evident to everyone that Sam could not get along with Joe and could not control his anger. The group was uncomfortable being in the same room with the two men. The director was forced to have Sam leave the program.

Any patient whose behavior adversely impacts other patients should be removed immediately from the program. Shouting, obvious agitation, or crying or prolonged sullen withdrawal will have a negative emotional impact on all the participants, not just upon the person who is the target. Hitting poses a real physical danger to other patients and even to the hitter.

Sue was capable of doing the program's activities but was incontinent. On the days when there were no field trips, the staff simply made certain she went to the toilet frequently. On the rare occasions when she soiled herself she changed her clothes. However, her incontinence was a problem on field trips. She frequently soiled herself before the staff could find a bathroom. Sue was embarrassed by her incontinence and by being removed from the group for extra toilet trips. She tried wearing adult diapers for a while, but still felt out of step with the other patients. Finally she stopped coming.

Incontinence is not a major issue for most early stage patients. However, it is an embarrassing issue for most of them. Constipation or the urgent need to urinate are common problems of the elderly, but not common subjects of discussion. Toilet times should be a regular and natural part of any early care program, without the need to place undue attention on bodily functions. When a patient must go to the toilet more often than other group members, frequently soils clothing, or must always be near a toilet, then it is appropriate to consider asking the patient to leave the group.

The patient who wanders is also a poor candidate for an early stage group. Even if the program is held in a locked unit and there is no chance the patient will slip away, wandering will be distracting to other patients.

The wanderer is a real problem on field trips or in unlocked units. Even a diligent staff will become exhausted by trying to keep the wanderer from harm while also meeting the needs of other group members.

> Jean always tried to wander from the group. She would edge slowly out of a group as she looked around for an exit. One day the group went on a field trip to a nature museum. The museum's major draw was a display of live raptors. A large hawk with a damaged wing sat on a perch on the main floor. Docents warned visitors to stay far away since the hawk, although tied to the post, had sharp talons and would lash out if approached. Jean was fascinated and kept trying to get near the bird.
>
> A staff member shadowed Jean during the entire field trip, but at one point while the docent was talking another patient stepped between the staff member and Jean. Jean used this as a chance to reach toward the hawk, but her grasp fell slightly short of the angry hawk's talons. After the trip the director removed Jean from the group for Jean's own safety.

It is appropriate to remove a patient from a group when:

- The patient's behavior has a negative emotional impact on other group members.
- The patient's behavior can cause physical harm to self or others.
- The patient is incontinent.
- The patient wanders.

IDENTIFYING THE CAUSE OF THE BEHAVIOR

Problem behavior can be a symptom of dementia or it can be caused by staff, another patient, or other factors.

Staff

The client with Alzheimer's disease has not lost basic emotions but has become slightly less adept at concealing them. As any normal person would, the early stage patient may dislike certain individuals, be fond of others, or simply choose to ignore an individual altogether.

Those attitudes will come to the fore readily in the first weeks of the program. A patient who dislikes a staff member will make an effort to sit at a distance from that person, will be unlikely to listen attentively to instructions by that staff member, and may, in fact, respond with outright animosity. If pressed to explain, the patient may be unable to do so or may even deny the feeling.

If staff size permits, this need not be an issue. The client should simply be paired with an individual who strikes a more responsive note. Trying to force the client to be friendly when those feelings are not real will not be productive.

However, sometimes the situation cannot be remedied. In that case, the client should leave the program.

Maggie was enrolled in a program by her nephew, her conservator. She lived in a group home where she was allowed to smoke, eat what she chose, and spend her days watching television. She had protested vigorously about coming to the program, particularly when told that smoking was not permitted.

At first the director paired off with Maggie. Maggie, an excellent mimic, mocked the director's flamboyant style and embarrassed the director. Unable to handle the situation, but hoping to keep Maggie in the program, the director paired her with a younger staff member.

Maggie withdrew and became monosyllabic. The young volunteer tried to get Maggie to take an active part in activities, but Maggie sat stolidly for hours. However, every time she could get away from the staff, she would try to smoke.

Other staff members tried to get Maggie interested in the program, but no one could. Staff members complained of the time and effort it took to keep Maggie from smoking. Reluctantly, the director told Maggie's nephew that Maggie had to leave the program.

On the other hand, the problem may be that a staff member does not like a patient. The staff member may find it easier to conceal the emotion, but eventually some incident may reveal the attitude. The staff member may avoid sitting with the patient, fail to call on the patient during group activities, or sometimes show annoyance or impatience.

Because of the intense one-on-one contact this type of program requires, it is not possible to brush over such incidents. The incident and feelings should be discussed in the staff meeting, and it may be that the staff person will have to leave the job.

Sometimes the issue may be the director's behavior. This can be awkward for other staff members, who may not know how to deal with a superior, may not be sure their own response is the preferable one, or may fear recrimination.

Occasionally the patients themselves will address the situation.

> Joan, a center director, never used straightforward language for toileting. "Now, let's all go tizzle," was her favorite euphemism. She always said this with a giggle and a slight flush. The staff disliked this intensely but no one knew what to say. They usually appeared not to hear the offending words and simply took the patients to the toilet.
>
> One day the oldest patient, Ann, spoke out. "What is all this tizzle, anyway? Why don't you ever just tell us you want us to go to the bathroom?"
>
> Startled, Joan mumbled, "What?"
>
> Not at all shy, Ann repeated herself. Thereafter Joan did not use the euphemism.

This was a mild problem, in any case, but other tougher issues can arise. A director can be patronizing, for example, or show favoritism to one or two patients, or withhold important information about a patient from the family so that the patient will stay in the program.

If the director's actions appear to be damaging the program, and the staff cannot speak directly to the director, then the staff should appeal to the board.

A common issue in any group is favoritism. Often the staff may not mean to choose favorites or might not even be aware of having done so. The staff should carefully monitor themselves and be certain that all patients are getting equal attention, responsibilities, and treatment. Staff should especially avoid making remarks about patients in front of other patients, such as, "Isn't that Peg just the sweetest thing?" If the group did like Peg before the remark, they might not after hearing it, or they might wonder why the staff doesn't say the same thing about them.

Typical behavioral problems can be caused by staff members. Among these are:

- The patient does not like a staff member and refuses to cooperate.
- A staff member does not like a patient and does not hide the attitude.
- The director is doing something wrong or inappropriate but no one challenges it.
- The staff shows favoritism.

Other Patients

Each patient will have a distinct personality, which, in early stage, will be relatively intact. However, certain traits may be exaggerated since the ability to control emotions and to respond to social settings is slightly impaired.

Among behaviors that may emerge are care-giving, competition, criticizing, monopolizing group time, and sullenness.

The woman who has been a caregiver all her life will want to care for people in the group. This can become annoying to other group members who neither seek nor want the attention.

Often the situation resolves itself naturally and amicably. For every caregiver there is usually someone who delights in receiving care. It is not uncommon for group members to pair off or form small subgroups of complementary personalities.

Occasionally this does not happen and the behavior becomes a problem. In that case it is important for the staff to give the caregiver tasks that will make her feel needed but will not involve other patients, such as folding the napkins for the lunch.

However, it is important to note that group members tend to compete for attention from the staff. If one patient is singled out for an activity such as folding napkins, other group members should be given tasks also, perhaps putting the tablecloth on the table or setting out plates. It is possible to eliminate one problem behavior without creating another.

Usually each group has a critical member who finds something wrong one way or another. When the target is the program or a specific activity, the staff can look deeper and determine whether the patient has a legitimate complaint that can be remedied. For example, perhaps the patient will be less critical of the outing if given a chance to choose the restaurant.

When the target is a staff member or another patient the issue cannot be handled as readily. The criticism can be personal and painful, such as criticizing someone's hairstyle, or merely provocative, such as criticizing the way someone slices an apple.

Rather than singling out an individual, the director should first talk with the group about being kind and then state outright that it is unacceptable to demean another person in the group. Sometimes the offender will continue to be critical and will obviously upset other patients. Then the director needs to have a private talk with the offender, explain the problem clearly, and say what the patient must do to stay in the program.

Generally each group will have a monopolizer—a patient who wants to dominate the conversations, has an opinion about everything, wants to be the first to do the activities, and usually does not know that the other patients are not impressed with this behavior.

The monopolizer can be a real problem for group dynamics. In many cases, the monopolizer may at first be a real charmer, breaking the ice with a funny story, or being willing to volunteer to sing or make the luncheon salad. Then it becomes evident that the monopolizer cannot get enough attention and will not yield the platform to anyone else. Other patients may give up and withdraw, become angry and resist the monopolizer's directions, or simply ignore the situation and try to carry on without attention.

In this case it is helpful for the staff to take the focus off the monopolizer by planning a range of activities in which all participate. For example, if the monopolizer loves to sing, do not plan an entire day filled with musical activities.

Or, if the monopolizer tries to dominate every conversation, the director should plan an activity where each person in the circle speaks in turn and thus has an equal chance to talk. This makes it possible for the director to avoid snubbing the monopolizer but to make it clear that everybody has a voice.

These same techniques work for the patient who is withdrawn. Staff members should not force a confrontation if a withdrawn patient does not want to take part in an activity. However, in a non-threatening situation where everyone is taking a turn, the withdrawn individual usually takes at least a small role.

Sullen behavior is a problem only if it is consistent. Everybody has a bad day at some point, and early care patients can have a bad day because of anything from constipation to medication to the onset of a new symptom of dementia.

If a patient is atypically uncooperative and peevish, staff should look for possible reasons for the behavior. The patient may well belong at home for the day and can rejoin the program as soon as the condition improves. However, if the patient is consistently brusque toward other patients, refuses to take part in any activity, or shows evident signs of wishing to be elsewhere, it is likely that the patient should leave the group.

Patients can sometimes interact in negative ways with other patients. This behavior can usually be countered with a simple change in daily activities.

- An obsessive caregiver can be assigned tasks to do for the whole group such as folding napkins.
- A critical patient can be given the chance to help plan activities or simply be told that personal criticism is demeaning and unacceptable.

- Activities should neither focus on a monopolizer nor exclude a withdrawn patient.
- Sullen behavior may be the result of illness or medication and is a problem only if consistent.

Other Factors

Medication, illness, and stress can cause behavior changes in anyone. For the Alzheimer's disease patient, any of those factors can produce marked changes.

> John, normally a cheerful man, sat somberly in the corner during the morning's activities. He picked at his lunch, leaving most of it uneaten. When a volunteer questioned him about how he was feeling, he snapped at her and told her to leave him alone.
> Puzzled by this change in John's mood, the director spoke to his daughter. The daughter explained that John had been nauseated for several days. His doctor had given him a drug which stopped the nausea but made John lethargic and temporarily reduced his appetite.
> Since John was no longer nauseated, his daughter had seen no reason to discuss the situation with the staff when she dropped John off in the morning. John was too reserved and embarrassed to tell anyone himself. The next week, when the side effects of the medicine were gone, John was his usual cheerful self.

Sometimes determining the problem can be as simple as discussing it with patient or caregiver. A constipated client may need more fluid intake; a diarrhetic one, to avoid fruit and salad.

A client may be taking a new drug that interacts with an old one and produces depression, nausea, or other side effects.

A client may have influenza and be tired, an earache and be disoriented, or a headache and be irritable.

Usually the client can discuss such illnesses or problems, but may not always do so. Older people sometimes consider such matters private, or may be embarrassed by what their bodies are doing.

The most difficult issue to discuss is a problem at home. Sometimes the problem is just a matter of communication. Habits and patterns change in the early stage. A family member may not know that the patient no longer wants to be called by a certain pet nickname. Or the patient may have developed an intense dislike for a former favorite food or activity.

There may even not be a real problem; it is possible that the dementia has progressed to the point that the patient can no longer grasp reality. The patient may believe the spouse stole the door keys when in fact the patient lost them. The the patient may suddenly become fearful of a spouse or old friend.

Or there can be real problems, ranging from verbal abuse to confining the patient to a bedroom or beating the patient.

It may be difficult for the staff to determine whether the patient is actually being harmed or is losing a grip on reality. A demented patient can sound lucid and be completely convincing. The patient can display bruises and insist he was beaten by his son when in fact he fell in his bathtub.

If there is good communication between the family and the director then they should be able to discuss the problem. If there is a reason to suspect abuse, however remote the possibility, the director should report specifics to the local elder abuse prevention authorities who will do an official investigation.

Many factors can contribute to behavioral changes.

- Elderly patients may be too embarrassed to report illnesses or problems with bodily functions but may exhibit atypical behavior instead.
- Patients affected by dementia may not be able to communicate with family members or may be having delusions.
- The patient may be abused.
- Good communication with family members can help identify contributing factors.

The Dementia Itself

If all other factors have been ruled out, then the patient is probably exhibiting the behaviors and symptoms characteristic of dementia. As noted, these symptoms are as varied and individual as the number of patients who have the disease. One patient may have a short attention span while another can sit for hours doing one activity. One patient may chatter all day while another barely utters a sentence.

The behaviors may have physical origins, such as the urgent need to toilet, or mental ones, such as momentary agitation. The problem may be loss of language or decreased social inhibitions.

The dementia of Alzheimer's disease cannot be reversed. However, some characteristic behaviors can be controlled or channeled constructively, particularly in the early stage.

SOME CHARACTERISTIC EARLY STAGE BEHAVIORS

The well-trained staff will not be disconcerted by characteristic early stage behaviors. Coping with such behaviors should not disrupt the daily program.

Urgent Need to Toilet

Incontinence becomes an issue in the late stages of the disease, when patients have no bowel or bladder control. Most early stage patients retain control and can readily relieve themselves in a timely and appropriate manner.

Post-menopausal women, however, do lose some bladder control and are prone to urinate easily, sometimes when sneezing, laughing, or moving suddenly. This may make toileting an urgent matter.

Elderly men and women become constipated if they do not get sufficient fluid intake. The full feeling can result either in sluggish behavior or a recurring need to try to eliminate the fecal matter.

Each program site should have a bathroom, and if both men and women are in the group, separate bathrooms are preferable. The bathrooms should be equipped for disabled users, with grip bars and wide entrances.

In a high-functioning group, the patients should be free to go to the bathroom when they need to go. In a locked unit no one need accompany the patient. A staff person, however, should check for problems if the patient remains in the bathroom for an unusually long time. In an unlocked unit, where a patient could wander outside, a staff person should accompany the patient to the bathroom. The staff person should avoid looking like a watchdog, by either using the facility or pretending to do so.

However, some patients may be too embarrassed to leave the group to go to the toilet even though they have a need. This can be handled in two ways. The person will usually exhibit some signs of distress, such as squeezing legs tightly together or surreptitiously fumbling at the crotch. In that case, the director can either call for a group toilet break or can, as soon as it will not be noticeable to the group, speak to the patient about the problem.

Even in a high functioning group the director should schedule frequent toileting breaks for the entire group, including the staff, certainly no less often than every two hours. This allows a shy person to do what is necessary and also safeguards against the kind of urgent situations that cause accidents.

Breaks should be scheduled for logical times such as just before going on field trips, just after meals, a short time after drink breaks, or when something stressful has happened.

Patients should drink plenty of fluids during the day's program, but not caffeinated drinks such as coffee or sodas. Caffeinated drinks not only agitate people but they also stimulate frequent urination. Drinking fluids will help control constipation. However, drinking excessive amounts of fruit juice will cause diarrhea, so other options such as water and herbal teas should be alternated with juice.

Most early stage patients do not need assistance with toileting and will be embarrassed if watched. Staff persons should intervene only if it is obvious that the patient is having trouble. However, obvious signs of trouble such as grunts, which can indicate constipation, or a foul odor, which can signal diarrhea, should be noted and discussed with either patient or family. An exceptionally pungent odor in urine can signal infections and should also be noted.

Even in the best of situations accidents can happen. If this is the case, minimize the incident. If the patient has a change of clothing, let the patient get clean and dry and return to the group when comfortable. If not, help the patient get as clean and dry as possible and have the caregiver come to get the patient.

Never point out the incident to other patients. If someone insists on pointing it out then acknowledge the accident but proceed then to another activity.

- Most early stage patients are not incontinent but do need regular toilet breaks.
- A patient with the urgent need to toilet may be too embarrassed to go but will exhibit the need and should be offered the option.
- A staff member should accompany the patients to the toilet and monitor what goes on, but should not be intrusive or obvious.
- Accidents should be treated promptly and without undue attention.

Momentary Agitation

Prolonged agitation is uncommon in the early stage, but a patient might occasionally become agitated. Usually an agitated patient just wants to get away from the group, and it is a good idea to allow this to happen until the cause can be identified and a solution undertaken.

A group activity can stimulate a bad memory, for example. The patient might have appeared to be enjoying a group discussion of weddings then suddenly start crying and try to run away. The patient might be remembering a deceased spouse. Since early stage patients also have minimal control of emotions it is likely that the grief and loneliness have suddenly become disproportionate and the patient cannot bear being with other people.

Or, the agitation may be triggered by a change in routine. One day a family member may be too busy to bring the patient to the center and instead sends the patient in a taxi. The patient may not understand this and think the family is sending them away permanently. The patient will be anxious about getting back home and uncertain whether the family still cares.

Or, the patient may be ill, taking a new medication, may not have gotten enough sleep, or may be nauseated or temporarily incontinent.

The staff should first take the patient to a quiet place where a private conversation can be conducted. Then the staff should try to get the patient to explain what is wrong. Sometimes this will happen and the patient will calm down after taking some time away from the group to let the medication wear off, to take a nap, or to perform some bodily function.

Sometimes it is helpful to review what was going on just before the outburst and to talk about it until the patient can voice the painful emotion. A skilled director, for example, would recall the discussion about weddings and wonder whether something about the patient's marriage was triggering the behavior. If the patient is able to express grief over a spouse's death, even if the death occurred many years earlier, the director should recognize and acknowledge the force of the emotion and offer support to the patient. Eventually the patient is likely to regain control.

Occasionally the staff members do not find out what triggered the outburst but the patient becomes engrossed in some other activity and calms down. If the patient is not extremely agitated and it appears that a change of activity will help, start a different activity with the group and watch the patient's reaction.

Sometimes no amount of talk or distraction will calm the patient down. The irrational patient will not be satisfied until the family member actually comes to the center and takes the patient home.

An irrational patient may be having delusions or hallucinations and be completely out of touch with reality. If that is the case the director should talk with the family to determine the cause of the delusions, or to suggest that the patient see a doctor if the cause is unknown.

- Generally an agitated person will calm down more readily if isolated from a group and given time to regain self-control.
- Bad memories can trigger uncontrollable emotions which agitate a patient.
- Medication, illness, and lack of sleep can all agitate a patient.
- A change in routine may frighten a patient.
- If reason and a calm empathetic approach do not calm the agitated patient then the patient may be having delusions or hallucinations and should see a doctor.

Failure to Remember Words

Even mild aphasia poses a communication challenge to the director and other staff members. It is not just that the patient cannot remember how to say something and so may have a hard time expressing feelings and attitudes, although this is certainly one issue. The aphasic patient also has a hard time understanding questions and directions. Even the best communicators quickly learn that they speak too rapidly, say too much, and don't repeat themselves often enough.

Staff members should use simple, short sentences with only one thought in each sentence. Presenting the aphasic patient with many options in one sentence confuses the patient. The patient will most likely respond with the last thing that was said rather than a true preference because the last option is the easiest one to remember.

Sometimes staff members become impatient and try to fill in words for the patient. This is unacceptable because the patient might want to say something entirely different. Even if the patient takes a long time, the staff member should wait for the patient to provide the words, or to indicate that a response is temporarily impossible.

Even if the patient fails to find words, the astute staff person can pick up non-verbal clues. Body language and voice tone actually may communicate more than words. An aphasic patient may not be able to identify spaghetti carbonara by name but can indicate enjoyment by eating heartily and smiling.

The staff members should remember that patients can pick up non-verbal language also. A director who taps a foot or stares at the ceiling while an aphasic patient struggles to find words is obviously impatient. That director should not be surprised if the patient cannot remember anything and becomes withdrawn.

A staff person should never force an aphasic patient to use written materials such as songbooks. Research indicates that aphasic patients can remember entire songs even when they cannot read the words to the same songs (Gates & Bradshaw, 1977). Forcing the issue may inhibit the patient to the degree that the patient will not sing at all.

Last, the physical arrangement of the room will have a direct impact on communication. Circular seating arrangements provide the maximum opportunity for everyone in the group to be able to see everyone else, but only if the circle is relatively small. If seats are in traditional rows the speaker must be placed so as to be clearly visible to everyone.

- Communicate in short, simple sentences. Aphasic patients become confused easily and cannot remember multiple options.
- Do not fill in thoughts for an aphasic patient because the patient may not have that thought.
- Body language and voice tone communicate as much or more than words.
- Physical room arrangement impacts communication.

Extreme Emotions

Early stage patients frequently have extreme emotional reactions which are either inappropriate or seemingly unrelated to what is going on. They may cry readily, long intensely for an idealized past, express deep love for near-strangers, or become angry at imagined slights.

> Nancy became acutely depressed when she learned that some-one she barely knew had died. She began reading the obituaries daily, talked incessantly about various ill friends, and inevitably cried at every session. Other group members began avoiding Nancy and complained to the director. The director finally had a private talk with Nancy and learned that she was worried about her own death. She was crying and depressed because she imagined her own death was imminent and was going to be tragic.

The director learned rather quickly that Nancy's grief was caused by fear and not by the death of an acquaintance. Not every overreaction has such an obvious cause or a sensible pattern. One week a patient may make sweeping declarations of love to a stranger and the next ignore the person completely. Erratic and inappropriate responses are a part of the dementia that the patient cannot control. Thus it is useless to try to talk the patient out of behaving a certain way and attempts to do so may worsen the behavior.

It is not appropriate for the staff to dismiss the emotion since the patient is feeling it and expressing it. However, the staff should not do anything to prolong the extreme reaction. It is enough to acknowledge the behavior and help the patient cope with it.

- Some extreme emotional responses mask other underlying emotions the patient cannot articulate.
- Staff should neither ignore nor prolong the emotional situation.

CONCLUSION

Although individual behavior varies widely, some general behavior is characteristic of early stage patients. These behaviors can be readily identified and addressed by a well-trained staff.

In some cases the behavior cannot be modified and a patient will have to leave the group. Any patient who consistently disrupts the group or poses a danger to self or others should leave the group. Referral to a doctor who can determine the presence of hallucinations or other factors may be appropriate.

Most problem behaviors can be modified or eliminated with minimum difficulty. However, the burden for making this happens falls largely on the staff. Staff may find themselves confronting their own prejudices, behaviors, or limitations as they work with problem patients.

Program Structure

7

A small number of programs hold joint meetings of family and patients. Most of these groups split at some point to cover separate agendas. The majority of programs either sponsor concurrent caregiver groups or refer families to outside family support groups.

Some programs focus entirely on therapy and are conducted by psychologists or psychiatrists. Others are primarily educational forums. A few function completely as social clubs. The majority include group discussions, social activities, and education.

The average meeting time is 4 hours, usually punctuated with a lunch break. Since early stage patients are most alert in the early part of the day, most programs begin by 10 A.M. Programs that are entirely educational or strictly therapeutic meet for shorter times and meeting times vary.

This chapter will (a) examine some therapeutic assumptions underlying early stage groups, (b) discuss activities such as reminiscence, music therapy, and exercise, and (c) emphasize the importance of community ativities and intergenerational involvement.

105

FAMILY SUPPORT GROUPS

The question of whether to sponsor a caregiver or family support group raises significant issues. There is no one correct answer. Program planners must decide if family and patients will meet jointly, and if so, for how long.

At least four programs hold joint meetings of family and patients: Early Stage Strategy Group, Denver, Colorado; Memory Problem Groups, Northampton, Massachusetts; Early Stage Memory Loss Program, Ann Arbor, Michigan; and Support Group for Early Stage Dementia Patients, Rochester, New York. These programs differ significantly in structure and goals.

The Northampton group was originally 12 couples who met in separate groups. The staff began conducting joint meetings when the patients showed diminished capacity. The nature of the meetings changed markedly. Patients were no longer able to follow the original program plan due to diminished capacity. The caregivers' discussions became more inhibited. The group is evaluating the program to determine whether the model will be continued.

By contrast, the Ann Arbor group conducts a new program twice yearly. The groups begin with joint meetings and then split. The program is tightly structured with specific content and time limits. Each program includes time for emotional support and group process for both family and patients.

The Denver group structures joint work with the explicit goal of making families and patients independent and interdependent. As the program progresses the two groups hold some separate meetings. This program is exceptionally well organized, following the goals and structure outlined in its own detailed manual.

There are obvious limitations in joint meetings of family and patients. As the Northampton program clearly illustrates, family members in a joint program do not receive the same emotional benefits as when their concerns are the sole focus of a group. The Northampton program is unique in joining the groups in the later stages of the program. Other groups have handled this problem by separating family and patients when new issues were raised and families and patients had different concerns needing separate support groups.

At least one program has concurrent support groups for family and patients. The Early Stage Memory Loss Program, Baltimore, Maryland, functions as a peer support group led by volunteer facilitators. Brief evening meetings are held twice monthly.

Coordinator Jane Goldstein notes that members form strong bonds and are reluctant to move on when patients reach a different level and must leave the program. The Baltimore program illustrates that it is difficult for caregivers to give up support once it is established. When patients enter advanced stages of dementia the needs of caregivers change. They must give more physical care, cope with greater loss, and often assume new responsibilities such as financial management. An early care support group for caregivers cannot and should not address these concerns. If a caregiver support group is part of the program, the director should be prepared to move the family into a new support group at the appropriate time.

Caregiver support groups reach various audiences. The Club, Philadelphia, Pennsylvania, requires caregivers to attend four educational sessions. The Early Stage Strategy Group, which has joint meetings, educates caregivers and encourages them to form their own support groups, including patients, after the training is complete. A Morning Out Club, San Diego, California, sponsors a monthly support group which is open to the community.

Some programs do not include a family support component. This does not mean that the program planners are unaware of the family's needs. These programs handle the issue of family support by referral to appropriate community groups. Too, most directors spend time individually counseling family members even when there is not a concurrent support group.

The Neuropsychiatric Institute, Los Angeles, California, will provide counseling for the caregiver at the clinic. The DRC Club, Walnut Creek, California, refers families to readily accessible support groups. At least one program, Granada Hills Community Hospital, Granada, California, supports families by providing patient referrals when the dementia worsens.

Family support is a concern for the early intervention program
even though the primary focus is the patient.

- Some programs sponsor family support groups while others
  offer referrals instead.
- Family support groups can include patients.
- The early stage caregiver support group should end when the
  patient enters a new stage of dementia.

THERAPY AND THE EARLY
INTERVENTION GROUP

Therapy may be the explicit goal of an early intervention
group, but it is more likely to be an implicit component. A few
programs have clearly articulated theoretical methods, but most
combine a variety.

Occasionally therapy is the sole purpose of a group. The
Neuropsychiatric Institute began its group to help newly diagnosed dementia patients cope with major depression and
suicidal ideation. The Institute interns now use a group therapy
model to help patients evaluate coping patterns. Clients are re-
ferred by the Neuropsychiatric Clinic and the Brentwood Veteran's Administration.

The Eastern Massachusetts Alzheimer's Association, Cambridge, Massachusetts, has several patient groups led by psychologists and psychiatrists who volunteer their professional
services. These professionals use Rational Emotive Therapy in
group settings. Patients are evaluated annually to assess whether
they continue to have the cognitive ability to take part in this kind
of group.

One program includes specific time for therapy in a broader
curriculum. The Granada Hills Community Hospital group has
one hour weekly of psychotherapy led by a psychologist. The
program bills health insurance for these services.

A program may describe itself as a support group, which

means that it may have therapeutic goals but is not led by a professional therapist. Among these are the Support Group for Early Onset Alzheimer's Patients, Orlando, Florida, the Baltimore program, and the Rochester program. The Orlando program is unique in that an early stage patient formed and leads the group. These programs are inexpensive or free, informal, and can be highly emotional depending on the facilitator's skills and goals.

Occasionally a program includes no specific therapeutic content. These groups usually designate themselves as activities programs because they focus on the social life of patients. These include A Morning Out Club, San Diego, California, and the Friends Club, Washington, D.C.

The Adult Activities Center, Costa Mesa, California, appears to be an activities program, but its director is explicit about his therapeutic goal. The program is based on milieu therapy and the goal is to maximize the patients' independence (Prather, 1993).

For the most part, however, programs operate within a broad framework of therapeutic theory. The gerontologists, social workers, nurses, and other professionals who lead the groups usually have a general idea about therapeutic models, but develop a style that incorporates many theories.

Among the theoretical assumptions that can be applied to work with early stage patients are those of the founder of therapy, Sigmund Freud. Freud (1924) described the classic progression of the patient during dynamic psychotherapy. To put it briefly, the patient feels cared about, has an emotional catharsis, increases self-esteem and builds defenses.

This progression is desirable in therapy with early-stage patients. The patient needs to adjust to change, regain mastery of self and environment, and begin mourning (Cath, 1982). The early care program achieves this by providing structure, support, and involvement in a validating group process (Maves & Schulz, 1985).

The process can occur in more than one way. For example, the goal of milieu therapy (Coons, 1978) is to maximize the patient's independence. All activities and interactions are structured to achieve that goal.

The Costa Mesa program includes activities which are as close to normal as possible for the patients' age range. The physical exercise component includes bowling, fishing, fitness regimes, and miniature golf. Patients attend college lectures, go to art museums, and tour historical sites. They do public service projects. No aspect of the patients' development is ignored.

Patients and caregivers report a high level of satisfaction with the program. Patients look forward to socializing with peers and depend less on family members for emotional support. Because they are encouraged to do as much as they are capable of doing, they become more confident of their ability to take care of themselves and handle self-care with relative ease and sophistication. Patients report an overall lift in mood as a result of the pleasant activities, and are better able to communicate with spouses and other family members.

Other programs incorporate the feelings group model (Van Wylen & Dykema-Lamse, 1990). In some cases the model is employed directly and the group focuses its discussion on the impact the disease has on their lives. In most cases the impact arises in the context of other activities and then the model is employed.

Feelings groups derive from I. D. Yalom's focus group model (1975), which centers on the patient's inability to sustain personal relationships and self-esteem.

In feelings groups, validation is extremely important. Everyone is introduced and everyone is included in the discussion. The group leader plays a major role in controlling the direction of the group, drawing out reluctant members and setting limits on effusive ones. In the latter case the patient is commended and supported for being emotive but is not allowed to become obsessive.

Within this context, group members begin to build trust and to reveal more about themselves and their responses to what is happening to them. They begin to understand that others have similar feelings. Over time they learn that they can either disagree with another member or feel deep empathy for someone else.

A therapist may use a variety of methods to draw out a patient. For example, if a patient has multiple impairments, the therapist can determine which sense the patient prefers, and use imagery reflecting that sense, to strengthen communication. If a patient communicates primarily with words related to sight, the therapist responds to the patient's contributions with the affirming words, "It looks like . . . "; if hearing, "It sounds like . . ."; and if touch, "How does that strike you?"

Group activities such as music therapy or reminiscence therapy can elicit strong emotional responses from participants. The feelings group model enables program directors to use these responses for benefit of both the emotional patient and the entire group.

> Mary had been a prolific letter writer, but lost her ability to remember words. The group was talking about Christmas when Mary remembered that she had been unable to send out Christmas cards. She began crying. The director used the opportunity to let members talk about their various losses. One other woman said she had the same problem, while others said they had thought they could still write until they tried to fill in forms at the doctor's office. The brief interaction in the day's activities provided major therapeutic benefits for all.

Each of these therapeutic methods in some way improves the patients' self-esteem, diminishes loneliness, and increases social skills.

* Some early care groups focus exclusively on activities.
* Theoretical bases are diverse and often mixed.
* Therapy in early stage programs is not expensive. When it is provided by professionals as a distinct service it is billed to insurance. Otherwise it is included in the fee package.

ACTIVITIES

Lindeman, Corby, Downing, and Sanborn (1991) identified five kinds of activities for demented patients: *physical, social, in-*

tellectual, functional, and *miscellaneous*. This model is readily applied to early-care programming.

Physical Activities

The benefit of physical activity has already been discussed. Men's groups are more apt to emphasize sports, such as bowling or miniature golf. A few groups offer dancing. The Costa Mesa group has access to fitness equipment and its members have supervised workouts using exercise bicycles, rowers, weights, and treadmills. Its members also take paced walks. Walking is the major exercise of several other groups.

Some groups, such as The DRC Club, modify a routine generally used in mid-stage day-care programs. Because the patients are elderly, disoriented, and generally fairly reserved about their bodies, the director will usually have the patient remain seated during the routine. Some patients may be more comfortable standing or seated on the floor at appropriate times during the routine.

Obviously the director should join in the routine, so that less cognizant patients can copy, but also to emphasize that the workout is pleasurable. The routine includes raising hands over heads, stretching both arms foreward, touching shoulders, rotating the head, putting the chin on the chest, extending legs, kicking legs up, placing feet flat on the floor, then taking deep breaths, and relaxing all the muscles.

This routine can last 10 minutes to a half hour, depending on number of repetitions and group ability. The emphasis is on gentle stretching, movement of all major muscle groups, and relaxation. Appropriate music can be played if desired.

If a patient is unable to do one of the movements or resists doing some part of the routine, do not make it an issue. If the workout is a struggle or frustrates the patient, then it will be counterproductive.

Generally the physical activities of the program should take no more than 1 hour of a 4-hour session. In some special sessions, when the major focus is the game, a longer time is acceptable.

Physical activities can take many forms.

- Men's groups take part in sports and structured workouts.
- Women may dance, walk, or do various exercises.
- Exercises should be relaxing, age-appropriate, and easy to understand.

Functional Activities

Functional activities are tasks such as grooming, toileting, cleaning, cooking, and eating. These activities receive far more emphasis in mid-stage day-care programs, because patients have less ability to do most of those tasks.

However, these tasks must still be done even in an early-care program. For the most part, this simply means being realistic about scheduling activities. Patients are able to dress themselves, comb their own hair, wash their own hands, and otherwise handle self-care, but they need extra time to do so. For example, taking adequate time to put on outerwear before an outing will lessen the chance that someone will go to the site without gloves or hat. Likewise, taking time before coming home will lessen the chance that items will be left behind and lost.

Toileting has been discussed previously. It is sufficient to note here that toilet breaks should be scheduled frequently and monitored adequately.

The most significant functional activity in the early care program is eating. Having lunch is one of the major activities of many groups. This can be a brown-bag event, the center can provide the meal, the group can make a potluck meal, or the group can go out to a restaurant. Each situation poses its own challenges.

If the meal is a brown-bag event, the director should give advance warning to the person who brings the patient to the meeting. The patient may well forget to bring a meal otherwise. As an earlier discussion indicated, someone should monitor the contents if the patient prepares the meal. Since something may happen with even the best planning, the director should have extra food available so that no one goes without lunch.

If the meal is a potluck, the same precautions apply. In addition, the potluck should not be unstructured; everyone should be assigned a specific item to bring. Preparing the meal together, each patient doing tasks according to skills, can be a satisfying group experience. The director and staff should assume responsibility for making the project work since patients are often confused about how to do the routine task of setting up meals. For example, one patient might chop fruit, another make sandwiches, a third set the table, and a fourth pour beverages. The director would be certain that everybody had a place setting, enough drinks were poured, and the food was arranged attractively on the table.

Meals are unlikely to be provided unless the sponsoring agency provides meals for participants in concurrent programs. It is unwise for early stage patients to eat with patients in later stages of dementia because they may begin to anticipate their own decline and become depressed.

Patients may go out to restaurants. In that case many factors should be considered. The director should first visit the restaurant to see whether facilities can adequately handle the group's needs. It is not necessary to have a separate room but the patients should not be crowded or seated in different parts of the restaurant.

The director should make arrangements with the manager so that the group does not have to wait upon arrival and seating is prompt. The food servers should be informed of the patients' limitations in advance. However, other diners should not be able to single out the group for undue attention. The goal is to help patients remain functioning members of society and this will be defeated if everyone in the restaurant stares.

The director should take a copy of the menu to the group. The group can then make decisions in advance about what they want to eat. Patients will be distracted by having made the trip to the restaurant, being in a new environment, and other people. The restaurant is not the place for patients to make decisions about what to eat.

The director must decide whether or not patients will make the actual order, however. Groups with high functioning members may prefer to place their own orders. Other groups may be content to let the director speak for them. If someone suddenly decides to change an order and it appears necessary, then do so, but do not precipitate a situation where everyone will change orders.

The director should collect money in advance. This will relieve the patient of worrying about tips or how much to spend. It will also avoid losses or theft.

The meal should proceed as normally as possible. Patients can ask for more water or whatever else they might need just as any other diner would. Staff members should seat themselves next to any patient needing extra help to eat and unobtrusively provide the help.

In addition to structured meals, most groups provide times for beverages and snacks. Obviously these should be nourishing and the staff members should monitor the amount and frequency of intake.

Functional activities are not a major concern of early care groups, but do have a certain role in the program. Functional activities will take a minimum of an hour and will take longer when there are trips.

- Adequate time should be allowed for self-care.
- Meals can be brown-bag events, potlucks, catered, or restaurant outings.
- Snacks and beverages should be monitored.

Cognitive Activities

Cognitive activities include jigsaw puzzles, a current events discussion, word games, and reminiscence. This is a very sensitive area because it is easy to choose an activity that will make one or more of the participants feel inadequate.

For example, a familiar word game is a completion exercise. The director begins a well known thought, such as, "A stitch in time . . ." A patient completes the thought with the words "saves nine."

This is not always easy. It poses a particular challenge if the group is multicultural. In one group a patient had neither been born nor educated in the United States. Her early training did not include memorizing familiar American aphorisms. She was still very alert and able to maintain her own household, but she could not complete the sentences. The director continued the exercise until the patient was humiliated by her failure.

This kind of insensitivity to varying skill levels can also create negative group dynamics. Another patient was very good at the game and repeatedly shouted out the answers. The director did nothing to stop her and even praised her for being so quick. The patient was thrilled at the recognition and talked about it all afternoon, completely oblivious to her peer's humiliation.

If cognitive activities are included then they should be structured so that everyone succeeds and attention is bestowed equally. If an activity is under way and does not meet that standard it should be terminated immediately.

A patient's skill level will be strongly influenced by cultural background, social class, ethnicity, education, and other factors that may not be readily apparent. The director should consider these underlying factors when a patient has difficulty with an activity. The difficulty may be more reflective of these factors than of the patient's abilities. The same person may excel at a more relevant cognitive test.

Cognitive activities should be limited to the amount of time that all participants can take part without failing.

- Cognitive activities should never embarrass or demean a patient.
- Patients will excel at different cognitive tests according to personal backgrounds.

Social Activities

Meals and meal preparation are actually one form of social activity. Others include singing, visits, parties, holiday celebrations, and reminiscence. Social activities reinforce familiar experiences and offer a change to enjoy interchanges with other people.

Visitors can be pets, children, or special people such as musicians, clowns, or actors. Having a visit enables the group to make special preparations for someone else, meet new and interesting people, and remember similar visits from other times in their lives.

Not everyone will be pleased with a pet visit. Some patients may fear animals or dislike their odor. If a patient does not wish to touch an animal or be near it, do not force the matter. It is best if the director or the person who brings the animal handles it. The animal will be frightened at the new place and new faces and could scratch or urinate. However, some opportunity for petting should be included.

Most patients really enjoy visiting with children. The person supervising the children should explain well ahead of the visit what Alzheimer's disease is and does, and prepare the children for the behavior they might expect. Most children will be sympathetic and not stare at the patients or mock them, but are likely to be curious no matter how well informed. Patients usually answer children's honest questions straightforwardly.

Usually the children present a short program or do something such as make tea for the patients. The patients seem to enjoy the attention and to applaud the efforts. Occasionally the two groups undertake tasks together, such as doing puzzles or crafts. In that case, the children may reinforce the patients' self-esteem by praising their work or helping them with difficult tasks.

Children are not unilaterally unreserved, but are generally more prone to openly express affection than are adults. They may hug the patients or shake their hands, usually smile broadly, and will exhibit good feelings readily. This uninhibited display of emotion and affection can be a positive boost for patients.

One other major social activity is reminiscence, which is also a cognitive activity. Patients discuss their past. This can be done informally, in brief periods, such as when someone mentions the first home they lived in, and everyone then talks about their first homes. Or it can be done in a systematic way using a life review (Taylor, van Amelsvoort, Jones, & Zeiss, 1983) or as reminiscence therapy (Head, Portroy, & Woods, 1990).

In the formal use of reminiscence, the leader helps the patients recall their life memories systematically. A topic of discussion is chosen and is the focus of the memories. Childhood memories include games, favorite toys, what they wanted to become, family stories, schools, and clubs. Their teenage memories may include first dates, first cars, and first jobs. Early adulthood focuses on career moves, marriage, first home, and having children. Later memories may focus on other jobs, achievements, vacations, and their children's growth.

In general, men tend to date their memories by concurrent historical events and women by what their children were doing at the time (Head, Portroy, & Woods, 1990). A man would recall that he got a job promotion on the day a president died, but a woman would recall the same event as the day her son had a fight at school.

Reminiscence helps the patient reinforce identity and maintain self-esteem. Recalling the past can restore a patient's sense of achievement, humor, or belief in love and joy. Conversely, if handled the wrong way, the process can trigger depression and lower self-esteem. It is critical for the director to use the exercise to convince the patient that he or she is still a worthy individual with many insights to offer to others.

Social activities also include outings, which can challenge the patients' cognitive and physical abilities, as well as social skills. These include trips to museums, gardens, lectures, beaches, movies, bookstores, and other sites that may interest the patients. These activities should be planned well in advance with the cooperation of any involved agency. Many museums and gardens have specially trained docents who will give the group a special tour and lead suitable activities.

The group should not go on the outing if the day is too hot, too cold, or the weather is completely inclement. The director should always have a backup plan in case this occurs.

The director should also make transportation arrangements well in advance of the event. Someone should be available for backup if a regular driver is ill or absent.

Social activities are the sole focus of some groups and the major focus of most. These will take a minimum of an hour.

- Social activities restore self-esteem and improve cognitive abilities.
- Reminiscence may be informal or highly structured.
- All social outings should include backup plans.

Miscellaneous Activities

Miscellaneous activities include art therapy, music therapy, and community service projects.

Art therapy can be enjoyable and productive. However, it can just as easily be the opposite. If patients are unable to do the craft they will feel inadequate. If the craft is too simple the patients will feel demeaned.

> A director hired an art teacher to come in for an afternoon and help patients make Thanksgiving centerpieces. The teacher came with an elaborate project involving cutting paper, painting, and using glue and glitter. The patients were hopelessly frustrated. Many could not measure the paper and ended up with sheets that were too big or too small. Some spilled paint on their clothing. Others could not keep up with the teacher. The staff tried to help slower patients, but the mess and errors increased when they did and tensions built between the staff members and patients. No one was happy.

When crafts projects are scheduled they should be simple and easy to complete. Everyone should be able to follow the directions, do their project alone, and complete something they can be pleased to take home.

However, the patient should not be forced to do a demeaning activity such as working in coloring books. The patient will feel he or she is being compared with a child. The activities should make use of the remaining skills even if those are limited.

Music remains a favorite activity even when the dementia advances. In the early stage, music therapy can actually help patients retain skills. Music therapy raises the patient's metabolic rate and reduces stress (Mazziotta, Phelps, Carson, & Kohl, 1988).

Music therapy can take a variety of forms. For example, music can be used with other activities, such as the exercise program described earlier in this chapter. Or, patients may make the music themselves using instruments such as the triangle. Patients may sing music which has a certain theme, such as music about rivers or horses. This can be accompanied by reminiscence therapy. Or patients may test their cognitive ability by trying to recall all the songs they remember that contain a certain word, such as red or blue or stars.

Finally, community service projects play a significant role in many programs. Patients can readily do volunteer work at many agencies. They are able to stuff envelopes and do many of the tasks that agencies are eager to have done by anyone who will.

Or a group may choose to take on a project for an agency, such as making an appropriate craft, assembling gift baskets, or a similar project that does not exceed the group's capacity.

Higher functioning patients will want to know something about the agency they are serving. It is appropriate for the group's director or the agency director to offer a simple explanation of the agency's program.

The patients will feel good about doing something for someone else. Also the patients will feel good about succeeding in a task, taking pride in how many envelopes were stuffed.

These activities usually take an hour of the sessions and can take more if accompanied by other activities such as reminiscence.

Art, music, and public service can all enhance a patient's self-esteem.

- Art projects should be neither too simple nor too complex.
- Music therapy enhances other skills.
- Community service helps patients believe they are still worthwhile to someone else.

CONCLUSION

The early stage group has the choice of a wide range of activities. Activities should be chosen with the program's specific goals in mind, whether those are therapeutic, social, or educational.

Sex, culture, class, and education can all play significant roles in whether a patient will benefit from an activity. Activities should be chosen with those factors in mind.

Every program should be structured with a backup plan. Each activity carries possibilities of problems, but most can be avoided with advance planning.

The director and staff members should have a clear agenda and stick to it. It is helpful to post the day's agenda in a visible place and have the group refer to it during the day.

The day should always begin with introductions and a check to see that everyone is prepared for the day's events. Each day should include times for breaks, movement and some quiet reflection. The day should end with a formal wrap-up and individual good-byes.

Closure

8

A number of issues arise when a patient is no longer a suitable member of an early intervention program. These include how to determine when that point has been reached, how to refer the patient to a more appropriate group, how to work with families, and how the staff members are to deal with their own feelings about the termination.

PATIENT TERMINATION ISSUES

Evidence that someone should leave a group is usually clear. The three most common reasons are incontinence, inability to follow directions because of increased aphasia, and signs that social control is slipping.

In some cases the issue of terminating patients is relatively easy. Many groups are time-limited and the program terminates automatically. No one has expectations about prolonged contact so termination is not an issue.

Occasionally a patient or family may understand that the patient can no longer handle group membership and will volun-

tarily opt out of the program. This can be emotional for all concerned but does not carry the same emotional weight as being
asked to leave.

Other programs slate specific breaks in the group cycle and
reevaluate each patient at those times. Typically these programs
operate for 6 to 10 weeks, then have a break. If a patient has
shown signs of deterioration then the patient is not asked back for
the next cycle of the group. This is less painful for the group as a
whole, since someone does not just abruptly leave the group.
However, it is still painful for the person who is asked to leave.

Other programs do not have hard rules about terminations and
may allow patients to stay even though they are not capable of
doing the activities. As the Northampton program illustrates, it is
not always the patients or family who prolong groups beyond the
reasonable time. Rather than ask members to leave, the directors
changed the program from concurrent meetings of family and
patients to joint meetings. As noted, although the program continued, family members became inhibited in voicing concerns.
The preferable solution would have been to ease the patients into
a day-care program more suited for their increased disability.

Referring a patient to a more suitable group is not as easy at it
might appear. It is not simply a matter of giving a list of day-care
programs to the family.

If the group has been explicit about naming and discussing the
disease, then the patient will know that it is time to move to the
next stage of care. This will not be easy, but the patient will
understand that it is necessary. This does not mean that denial,
anger, and grief will not surface in the termination process. To the
contrary, these behaviors are likely to intensify.

If the group has been primarily a social group or has minimized
discussion of issues, then the patient will not want to give up
friends and happy activities. A new program with limited activities will seem unsuitable and the patient is unlikely to cooperate.

Even if a day-care program is found, the family may be shocked
by the rapid decline in the patient's condition. Without the
stimulation of more able peers and challenging activities, the
patient may decline. The patient, asked to throw a large ball back

and forth or color a picture, may rapidly lose self-esteem. Or the patient may become more agitated when exposed to other patients who wander or have delusions.

FAMILY TERMINATION ISSUES

Day-care programs function very differently from early intervention programs. Day-care programs are generally licensed, often entail medical intervention, and may be prohibitively expensive. Waiting lists are often long. Patients are readily dismissed if such behaviors as hitting or shouting emerge.

Families must negotiate an entirely new contract and this one is much more formal. Families may be neither able to cope with the sudden change in the way the patient is treated nor the financial demands.

It is a major adjustment for a family when a patient enters a new phase of the dementia. The physical demands increase, the patient becomes more irrational, and the prospect of death seems more real.

The family will try to delay this phase as long as possible. While the patient is enrolled in an early intervention program the family can maintain the illusion that the patient may recover. This is not the case when the patient enters day-care.

It is not uncommon for the family to become angry at the director and to accuse him or her of misjudging the patient's capabilities. The family may also plead for the director to reconsider, and in some instances may be successful.

Or, the family may become extremely dependent on the director, asking for emotional support as they lose their loved one. They may cry when they drop off or pick up the patient, may spend a long time detailing their problems, and are likely to repeat this for many weeks unless the director puts a speedy end to it.

It is important for the director not only to refer the patient to a day-care program but also to refer the family to a new support group. Many families will insist they have already confronted the issues and do not need to do so in yet another setting, but, as noted, the issues are different when the patient gets worse.

It will also be appropriate for the director to give the family lists of other places they can find help, such as respite services, the ombudsman, and social workers. Even if the director has already given the family the lists in the past it is useful to offer a list again.

STAFF TERMINATION ISSUES

Staff members are seldom prepared for the emotional wrench of terminating a patient. The sustained intimate contact with the patients builds the bond in invisible ways and the strength of the bond is suddenly visible when it is about to be broken. The staff members should prepare for this to happen and deal with it immediately. Prolonging the termination is not fair to the patient.

However, staff members should let the patient know that the experience has been important and that the decision to have them move on is hard. Being brusque to avoid feeling the emotional pain will only hurt the patient.

Staff members should not make false promises to stay in touch with the patient, to be a good friend, or to do anything that they are not going to do. If even the remote possibility exists that a promise will be broken then it should not be made.

Staff members may also have to cope with guilt, particularly if the family continues to have problems and tries to get the staff involved in solving them. If a patient fails in a day-care program the family may call the early intervention program director for sympathy. The staff members must distance themselves from the patients once the bond is broken.

Beyond these concerns, certain administrative concerns will arise. The staff must be able to recruit new members to replace the old ones. Sometimes all the group members will be new and there will be no problem with group unity. Other times the director will need to introduce one or two new members to an established group. The staff needs to have a plan for handling the questions of the old members, for making the new members feel welcome, and for maintaining group unity.

It is inevitable that staff members will make mental comparisons of old and new patients. These should never be voiced to the patients, who may perceive them as value judgments and will wonder why they do not measure up to the old patients.

The staff must also be prepared to deal with burnout. Someone may start out enthusiastically and become disillusioned by the time the third group begins meeting. Or someone else may simply be tired and unable to do the job. Vacations and time off should be maintained. If the group has distinct cycles or is time-limited, taking an extended break between the cycles or next group is advised. If not then the breaks should be scheduled routinely.

CONCLUSION

A well-designed program includes consideration of the emotional and practical issues of termination. These include meeting the needs of family, patients, and caregivers.

Bibliography

Altman, H. J. (Ed.) (1986). *Alzheimer's disease and dementia: Problems, prospects and perspectives.* New York: Putnam.

Baddeley, A. D. (1990). *Human memory: Theory and practice.* Hillside, NJ: Erlbaum.

Blair, S. N., Brill, P. A., & Kohl, H. W. (1989). "Physical Activity Patterns in Older Individuals." In W. W. Spriduso & H. M. Eckert (Eds.), *Physical activity and aging.* Champaign, IL: Human Kinetic Books.

Blessed, G., Tomlinson, B., & Roth, M. (1968). The association between quantitative measures of dementia and senile changes in the cerebral grey matter of elderly subjects. *British Journal of Psychiatry, 114,* 797–811.

Brawley, E. (1992). Alzheimer's disease: Designing the physical environment. *American Journal of Alzheimer's Care and Related Research, 7(1),* 3–8

Brechling, B., & Schneider, C. (1993). Preserving autonomy in early stage dementia. *Journal of Gerontological Social Work, 20,* 17–33.

Bright, R. (1988). *Music therapy and the dementias.* St. Louis: Magna Music.

Brody, E. M. (1985). Parent care as a normative family stress. *Gerontologist, 25,* 19–29.

Brookdale Foundation (1987). *How to start a respite service for people with Alzheimer's and their families.* New York: Brookdale Center on Aging, Hunter College, CUNY.

129

Brown, R., & Kulik, J. (1977). Flashbulb memories. *Cognition, 5,* 73–99.

Burns, A., Jacoby R., & Levy, R. (1991). Progression of cognitive impairment in Alzheimer's disease. *Journal of the American Geriatric Society, 39,* 39–45.

Cath, S. H. (1982). Psychoanalysis and psychoanalytic psychotherapy of the older patient. *Journal of Geriatric Psychiatry, 15,* 43–53.

Clemmer, W. (1992). *Victims of dementia.* Binghamton, NY: Haworth Press.

Cohen, D. (1991). The subjective experience of Alzheimer's disease: The anatomy of illness as perceived by patients and families. *American Journal of Alzheimer's Care and Related Disorders and Research, 6*(5), 128–133.

Coons, D. (1978). Milieu therapy. In W. Reichel (Ed.), *Clinical aspects of aging.* Baltimore: Williams & Wilkins.

Cooper, D. (1984). Group psychotherapy with the elderly: Dealing with life and death. *American Journal of Psychotherapy, 38,* 203–215.

Cummings, J. L., & Benson, D. F. (1986). Dementia of the Alzheimer type: An inventory of diagnostic clinical features. *Journal of the American Geriatrics Society, 34,* 12–19.

David, P. (1991). Effectiveness of group work with the cognitively impaired older adult. *American Journal of Alzheimer's Care and Related Disorders and Research, 6*(7), 10–16.

Drickamer, M. A., & Lachs, M. S. (1991). Should patients with Alzheimer's disease be told their diagnosis? *New England Journal of Medicine, 326,* 947–951.

Early Birds Support Group Summary. (1991). Honolulu Chapter of the Alzheimer's Association. Unpublished manuscript.

Feil, N. (1989). Validation: An empathetic approach to the care of dementia. *Clinical Gerontologist, 8*(3), 89–94.

Folstein, M. F., Folstein, S. E., & McHugh, P. R. (1975). Mini Mental State: A practical method for grading the cognitive state of patients for the clinician. *Journal of Psychiatric Research, 12,* 189–198.

Freud, S. (1989). *The Freud Reader.* Peter Gay (Editor). NY: W. W. Norton.

Gates, A., & Bradshaw, J. L. (1977). The role of the cerebral hemispheres in music. *Brain and Language, 4,* 403–431.

Goldstein, M. K., Gwyther, L. P., Lazaroff, A. E., & Thal, L. J. (1991). Managing early Alzheimer's care. *Patient Care,* Nov. 15, 44–48.

Goodglass, H., & Kaplan, E. (1972). *The assessment of aphasia and related disorders*. Philadelphia: Lea and Febiger.

Gwyther, L. P. (1985). *Care of Alzheimer's patients: A manual for nursing home staff*. Chicago: American Health Care Association and Alzheimer's Disease and Related Disorders Association.

Haggarty, A. D. (1990). Psychotherapy for patients with Alzheimer's disease. *South Florida Institute for Alzheimer's Disease Education and Research U.S. Advances.* Spring 1990, 55–60.

Harper, S., & Lund, D. A. (1990). Wives, husbands and daughters caring for institutionalized and non-institutionalized dementia patients; Toward a model of caregiver burden. *International Journal of Aging and Human Development, 30*(4), 241–262.

Hart, S., & Sample, J. (1990). *Neuropsychology and the dementias*. London: Taylor & Francis.

Haycox, J. A. (1984). A simple, reliable clinical behavioral scale for assessing demented patients. *Journal of Clinical Psychiatry, 141,* 1356–1364.

Head, D. M., Portroy, S., & Woods, R. T. (1990). Reminiscence: Is it worthwhile? *Journal of Geriatric Psychiatry, 5,* 295–302.

Hughes, C. P., Berg, L., Danziger, W., Coben, L. A., & Martin, R. L. (1982). A new clinical scale for the rating of dementia. *British Journal of Psychiatry, 140,* 566–572.

Krishnan, K. R., Heyman, A., Ritchie, J. C., Utley, C. M., Dawson, D. V., & Roger, H. (1988). Depression in early onset Alzheimer's disease. *Biological Psychiatry, 248,* 937–940.

Kubler-Ross, E. (1969). *On death and dying*. New York: Macmillan.

Lawton, M.P. (1982). Competence, environmental press and the adaptation of older people. In *Aging and the environment*. New York: Springer.

Lieb, R. (1982). How to buy chairs. *American Health Care Association Journal,* July, 21–24.

Lindeman D., Corby, N., Downing, R., & Sanborn, B. (1991). *Alzheimer's day care: A basic guide*. Washington, DC: Hemisphere Publishing.

Lindenmuth, G. F., & Moore, B. (1990). Improving the cognitive abilities of elderly Alzheimer's patients with intensive exercise therapy. *American Journal of Alzheimer's Care and Disorders and Related Research, 5*(1), 31–33.

McKhann, G., Drachman, D., Folstein, M., Katzman, R., Price, D., & Stadlan, E. M. (1984). Clinical diagnosis of Alzheimer's disease:

Report of the NINCDS-ADRDA Work Group under the auspice of Department of Health and Human Services Task Force or Alzheimer's Disease. *Neurology, 34,* 359–364.

Maves, R., & Schulz, J. W. (1985). Inpatient group treatment on short term acute care units. *Hospital and Community Psychiatry, 35,* 69–73.

Mazziotta, J. C., Phelps, M. E., Carson, R., & Kohl, D.E. (1988). Tomographic mappings of human cerebral metabolism: Auditory stimulation. *Neurology, 32*(9), 921–937.

Mesulam, M. (1987). Primary progressive aphasia—Differentiation from Alzheimer's disease. *Annals of Neurology, 22,* 533–534.

Morris, J. C., McKeel, D. W., Jr., Fulling, K., Torack, R. M., & Berg, L. (1988). Validation of clinical diagnostic criteria for Alzheimer's disease. *Annals of Neurology, 24,* 17–22.

Morris, R., & Kopelman, M. (1986). Memory deficits in Alzheimer-type dementia; A review. *Quarterly Journal of Experimental Psychology, 38a,* 575–603.

Perlmuter, L. C., Tenney Y., & Smith, P. (1980). *The evaluation and remediation of memory problems in the aged.* Boston: Veteran's Administration Outpatient Memory and Learning Clinic.

Prather, S. (1993). *Men's activity group for early diagnosed Alzheimer's patients and their families.* Unpublished manuscript.

Reisberg, B., Ferris, S. H., DeLeon, M. J., & Crook, (1982). The Global Deterioration Scale for Assessment of Primary Degenerative Dementia. *American Journal of Psychiatry, 139,* 1136–1139.

Riley, K. (1991). *Planning and implementation of support groups for Alzheimer's patients.* Unpublished paper, presented at 1991 Annual Scientific Meeting of the Gerontological Society of America.

Riley, K., & Carr, M. (1989). Group psychotherapy with older adults: The value of an expressive approach. *Psychotherapy, 26,* 366–371.

Rosen, W. G., Mohs, R. C., & Davis, K. L. (1984). A new rating scale for Alzheimer's disease. *American Journal of Psychiatry, 141,* 1356–1364.

Roth, M., Tym, E., Mountjoy, C. Q., et al. (1986). CAMDEX: A standardized instrument for the diagnosis of mental disorder in the elderly with special reference to the early detection of dementia. *British Journal of Psychiatry, 149,* 698–709.

Shephard, R. J. (1987). *Physical activity and aging.* London: Cambridge University Press.

Strang, V., & Neufeld A. (1990). Adult day care programs: A source for respite. *Journal of Gerontological Nursing, 16*(11), 16–20.

Taylor, S., van Amelsvoort, W., Jones, G., & Zeiss, E. (1983). Collecting and conducting life reviews. *Proceedings of the 1st Annual Gerontological Nurses Association, 2,* 114–118. Victoria, British Columbia, Canada.

Stevenson, J. P. (1990). Family stress related to home care of Alzheimer's disease patients and implication of support. *Journal of Neuroscience Nursing, 22*(3), 179–188.

10 physical reasons you may be depressed (1992). *Prevention,* June, 69–76, 134.

Teri, L.. & Reifler, B. V. (1987). Depression and dementia. In L. Carstensen & B. Edlestein (Eds.) *Handbook of clinical gerontology.* New York: Pergamon Press.

Tierney, M. C., Fisher, R. H., Lewis, A. J., et al. (1988). The NINCDS–ADRDA Work Group Criteria for the Clinical Diagnosis of Probable Alzheimer's Disease: A clinicopathologic study of 57 cases. *Neurology, 38,* 359–364.

Tully, M., & Turner, J. (1992). *Join the club: Meeting the special needs of men with Alzheimer's disease.* Greater Washington, D.C. Chapter of the Alzheimer's Association.

U.S. Congress, Office of Technology Assessment. (1987). *Losing a million minds: Confronting the tragedy of Alzheimer's disease and other dementias.* Washington, DC: Government Printing Office.

Van Wylen, M., & Dykema-Lamse, J. (1990). Feelings group for adult day care. *Gerontologist, 30*(4), 557–559.

Wylie, D. (1993a). *Descriptions of programs for high functioning dementia patients.* Unpublished manuscript.

Wylie, D. (1993b). *Chapters to contact regarding early stage patient programming.* Unpublished manuscript.

Yalom, I. (1975). *The theory and practice of group psychotherapy.* New York: Basic Books.

Yalom, I. (1983). *Inpatient group psychotherapy.* New York: Basic Books.

Zarit, S. H., Zarit, J., & Reeves, K. (1982). Memory training for severe memory loss: Effects on senile dementia patients and their families. *Gerontologist, 22*(4), 373–377.

Zgola, O. M., & Coulter, L. G. (1988). I can tell you about that: A therapeutic group program for cognitively impaired persons. *American Journal of Alzheimer's Care and Related Disorders and Research, 3*(6), 17–22.

Appendix A
Programs for High-Functioning Dementia Patients*

CALIFORNIA

Diablo Respite Center, The DRC Club, Walnut Creek, CA. 510–210–6196.

Granada Hills Community Hospital, CARE Club, Granada Hills, CA. 818–366–1967.

Neuropsychiatric Institute, UCLA, Los Angeles, CA. 310–825–0089.

San Diego Alzheimer's Association, A Morning Out Club, San Diego, CA. 619–295–2509.

South Coast Institute of Applied Gerontology, The Adult Activities Center, Costa Mesa, CA. 714–548–9331.

University of California, San Francisco, Support Groups for Newly Diagnosed Early Stage Alzheimer's Patients, San Francisco, CA. 415–673–3881.

*From David Wylie, "Descriptions of Programs for High Functioning Dementia Patients," 1993 unpublished paper. Reprinted by permission of the author.

COLORADO

Denver Alzheimer's Association, Early Stage Strategy Group, Denver, CO. 303–733–1669.

DISTRICT OF COLUMBIA

Greater Washington, D.C. Alzheimer's Association, Friends Club, Washington, D.C. 202–483–3310.

FLORIDA

Greater Orlando Alzheimer's Association, Support Group for Early Alzheimer's Patients, Orlando, FL. 407–422–9595.

HAWAII

Honolulu Alzheimer's Association, Early Birds Support Group, Honolulu, HI. 808–521–3771.

IOWA

Quad Cities Alzheimer's Association, Davenport, IA. 319–324–1022.

KENTUCKY

Lexington/Bluegrass Alzheimer's Association, The Lunch Bunch: A Support Group for Mild Memory Disabled Persons, Lexington, KY. 606–252–6282.

MARYLAND

Baltimore/Central Maryland Alzheimer's Association, Early Stage Memory Loss Program, Baltimore, MD. 410–435–4933.

MASSACHUSETTS

Eastern Massachusetts Alzheimer's Association, Cambridge, MA. 617–494–5150.
Western Massachusetts Alzheimer's Association, Memory Problem Groups, Northampton, MA. 413–586–5325.

MICHIGAN

Detroit Alzheimer's Association, Patient Support Group, Southfield, MI. 313–557–4742.
South Central Michigan Alzheimer's Association, Early Stage Memory Loss Program, Ann Arbor, MI. 313–741–8200.

NEW YORK

New York City Alzheimer's Association, Support Group for Early Dementia Patients, New York City, NY. 212–983–0700.
Rochester Alzheimer's Association, Support Group for Early Stage Dementia Patients, Rochester, NY. 716–442–3820.

OHIO

Cleveland Alzheimer's Association, Cleveland, OH. 216–721–8457.

OREGON

Columbia Willamette Alzheimer's Association, Portland, OR. 503–229–7115.

PENNSYLVANIA

Greater Philadelphia Alzheimer's Association, The Club, Philadelphia, PA. 215–568–6430.

Appendix B
Health Screening Program*

Patient's Name: _____

Date: _____

Instructions: *Ask the patient these questions and then check the appropriate answer.*

Have you had any of these problems in the past 12 months? Do you have them now?

	No	Yes	Now
Headaches			
Confused feeling			
Forgetful			
Trouble remembering			
Hard to concentrate			
Tired feeling			
Frequent weak feeling			
Trouble sleeping			

---

*From the Honolulu Chapter of the Alzheimer's Association. "Early Birds Support Group Summary," 1991 unpublished paper. Reprinted by permission of the Honolulu Chapter.

	No	Yes	Now
Trouble with appetite			
Sexual trouble			
Loss of 8 or more pounds			
Hard to breathe			
Hard to talk			
Tense, nervous			
Sad, depressed			
Lonely			
Angry, frequently mad			
Guilty			
Bad dreams			
Hopeless			
Helpless			
Scared			
Panic attacks			
Suicidal thoughts			
Can't stop thinking			
Suspicious			
Moody			
No friends			
Life is too much			
No job			
Empty feeling			

Appendix C
Mini-Mental State Exam*

Patient's Name _____

Examiner's Name _____

Date_____

ORIENTATION

10 (   ) What is the (year) (season) (date) (day) (month)? *Ask each question in turn. 1 point for each correct answer.*
Where are we: (state) (county) (town) (hospital) (floor). *Ask each question in turn. 1 point for each correct answer.*

REGISTRATION

3 (   ) *Ask the patient if you may test his memory. Then say the names of 3 unrelated objects, slowly and clearly. The first repetition determines the score, but repeat up to 6 trials.*

From Folstein, M.R., Folstein, S. E., & McHugh, P.R. (1975). Mini Mental State: A practical method for grading the cognitive state of patients for the clinician. *Journal of Psychiatric Research, 12,* 196–198. Reprinted with kind permission from Elsevier Science Ltd., The Boulevard, Langford Lane, Kidlington 0X5 1GB, UK.

ATTENTION AND CALCULATION

5 ( ) Serial 7's. *Ask the patient to begin with 100 and count backwards by 7. Stop after 5 subtractions. The score is the number right. If the patient cannot or will not then ask the patient to spell "world" backwards instead. The score is the number of letters in correct order.*

RECALL

3 ( ) *Ask the patient to recall the 3 objects in the registration sequence. Give 1 point for each answer.*

LANGUAGE

9 ( ) Naming: *Show the patient a watch and ask the patient to name the object. Do the same with a pencil. 1 point for each.*
Repetition: *Ask the patient to repeat the following:* "No ifs, ands, or buts." *1 point.* 3-stage command: *Hand the patient a blank piece of paper. Instruct the patient,* "Take a paper in your right hand, fold it in half, and put it on the floor." *1 point for each correct part.*
Reading. *On a blank piece of paper print the words* "Close your eyes." *Ask the patient to read it and do what it says. 1 point only if the patient closes eyes.*
Writing. *Give the patient a blank piece of paper and ask him to write a sentence. It must contain a subject and verb but grammar and punctuation need not be correct. 1 point.*
Copying. *Give the patient a picture of intersecting pentagons and ask the patient to copy it. The patient must draw 10 angles with at least 2 intersecting to score the point.*

___ TOTAL SCORE
Assess level of consciousness along a continuum and circle the appropriate word:
Alert   Drowsy   Stupor   Coma

Appendix D
Durable Power of Attorney for Health Care Decisions*

California Medical Association

DURABLE POWER OF ATTORNEY FOR HEALTH CARE DECISIONS

(California Civil Code Sections 2410- 2444)

WARNING TO PERSON EXECUTING THIS DOCUMENT

This is an important legal document. Before executing this document, you should know these important facts:

This document gives the person you designate as your agent (the attorney-in-fact) the power to make health care decisions for you. Your agent must act consistently with your desires as stated in this document or otherwise made known.

Except as you otherwise specify in this document, this document gives your agent power to consent to your doctor not giving treatment or stopping treatment necessary to keep you alive.

Notwithstanding this document, you have the right to make medical and other health care decisions for yourself so long as you can give informed consent with respect to the particular decision. In addition, no treatment may be given to you over your objection, and health care necessary to keep you alive may not be stopped or withheld if you object at the time.

This document gives your agent authority to consent, to refuse to consent, or to withdraw consent to any care, treatment, service, or procedure to maintain, diagnose, or treat a physical or mental condition. This power is subject to any statement of your desires and any limitations that you include in this document. You may

state in this document any types of treatment that you do not desire. In addition, a court can take away the power of your agent to make health care decisions for you if your agent (1) authorizes anything that is illegal, (2) acts contrary to your known desires or (3) where your desires are not known, does anything that is clearly contrary to your best interests.

This power will exist for an indefinite period of time unless you limit its duration in this document.

You have the right to revoke the authority of your agent by notifying your agent or your treating doctor, hospital, or other health care provider orally or in writing of the revocation.

Your agent has the right to examine your medical records and to consent to their disclosure unless you limit this right in this document.

Unless you otherwise specify in this document, this document gives your agent the power after you die to (1) authorize an autopsy, (2) donate your body or parts thereof for transplant or therapeutic or educational or scientific purposes, and (3) direct the disposition of your remains.

If there is anything in this document that you do not understand, you should ask a lawyer to explain it to you.

144

1. CREATION OF DURABLE POWER OF ATTORNEY FOR HEALTH CARE

By this document I intend to create a durable power of attorney by appointing the person designated below to make health care decisions for me as allowed by Sections 2410 to 2444, inclusive, of the California Civil Code. This power of attorney shall not be affected by my subsequent incapacity. I hereby revoke any prior durable power of attorney for health care. I am a California resident who is at least 18 years old, of sound mind, and acting of my own free will.

2. APPOINTMENT OF HEALTH CARE AGENT

(Fill in below the name, address and telephone number of the person you wish to make health care decisions for you if you become incapacitated. You should make sure that this person agrees to accept this responsibility. The following may not serve as your agent: (1) your treating health care provider; (2) an operator of a community care facility or residential care facility for the elderly; or (3) an employee of your treating health care provider, a community care facility, or a residential care facility for the elderly, unless that employee is related to you by blood, marriage or adoption. If you are a conservatee under the Lanterman-Petris-Short Act (the law governing involuntary commitment to a mental health facility) and you wish to appoint your conservator as your agent, you must consult a lawyer, who must sign and attach a special declaration for this document to be valid.)

I, _____, hereby appoint:

(*insert your name*)

Name _____

Address _____

Work Telephone (_____) _____   Home Telephone (_____) _____

as my agent (attorney-in-fact) to make health care decisions for me as authorized in this document. I understand that this power of attorney will be effective for an indefinite period of time unless I revoke it or limit its duration below.

(Optional) This power of attorney shall expire on the following date: _____.

© California Medical Association 1992 (revised)

California Medical Association. "Durable Power of Attorney for Health Care Decisions," Copyright 1992 by the California Medical Association. Reprinted by permission of the Association.

3. AUTHORITY OF AGENT

If I become incapable of giving informed consent to health care decisions, I grant my agent full power and authority to make those decisions for me, subject to any statements of desires or limitations set forth below. Unless I have limited my agent's authority in this document, that authority shall include the right to consent, refuse consent, or withdraw consent to any medical care, treatment, service, or procedure; to receive and to consent to the release of medical information; to authorize an autopsy to determine the cause of my death; to make a gift of all or part of my body; and to direct the disposition of my remains, subject to any instructions I have given in a written contract for funeral services, my will or by some other method. I understand that, by law, my agent may not consent to any of the following: commitment to a mental health treatment facility, convulsive treatment, psychosurgery, sterilization or abortion.

4. MEDICAL TREATMENT DESIRES AND LIMITATIONS (OPTIONAL)

(Your agent must make health care decisions that are consistent with your known desires. You can, but are not required to, state your desires about the kinds of medical care you do or do not want, including your desires concerning life-sustaining treatment. If you do not want your agent to have the authority to make certain decisions, you must write a statement to that effect in the space provided below; otherwise, your agent will have the broad powers to make health care decisions for you that are outlined in paragraph 3 above. In either case, it is important that you discuss your health care desires with the person you appoint as your agent.

(Following are three general statements about withholding and removal of life-sustaining treatment. If, after carefully reading all of these statements, you agree with one of them, you may initial that statement. If you wish to add to one of the printed statements, or to write your own instead, you may do so in the space provided.)

I do **not** want efforts made to prolong my life and I do **not** want life-sustaining treatment to be provided or continued: (1) if I am in an irreversible coma or persistent vegetative state; or (2) if I am terminally ill and the application of life-sustaining procedures would serve only to artificially delay the moment of my death; or (3) under any other circumstances where the burdens of the treatment outweigh the expected benefits. I want my agent to consider the relief of suffering and the quality as well as the extent of the possible extension of my life in making decisions concerning life-sustaining treatment.

If this statement reflects your desires, initial here: _____

I want efforts made to prolong my life and I want life-sustaining treatment to be provided **unless I am in a coma or persistent vegetative state** which my doctor reasonably believes to be irreversible. Once my doctor has concluded that I will remain unconscious for the rest of my life, I do not want life-sustaining treatment to be provided or continued.

If this statement reflects your desires, initial here: _____

146

I want efforts made to prolong my life and I want life-sustaining treatment to be provided **even if** I am in an irreversible coma or persistent vegetative state.

If this statement reflects your desires, initial here: _____

Other or additional statements of medical treatment desires and limitations: _____

_____

(You may attach additional pages if you need more space to complete your statements. Each additional page must be dated and signed at the same time you date and sign this document.)

5. APPOINTMENT OF ALTERNATE AGENTS (OPTIONAL)

(You may appoint alternate agents to make health care decisions for you in case the person you appointed in Paragraph 2 is unable or unwilling to do so.)

If the person named as my agent in Paragraph 2 is not available or willing to make health care decisions for me as authorized in this document, I appoint the following persons to do so, listed in the order they should be asked:

First Alternate Agent: Name _____   Work Telephone (_____) _____

Address _____   Home Telephone (_____) _____

Second Alternate Agent: Name _____   Work Telephone (_____) _____

Address _____   Home Telephone (_____) _____

6. USE OF COPIES

I hereby authorize that photocopies of this document can be relied upon by my agent and others as though they were originals.

DATE AND SIGNATURE OF PRINCIPAL
(You must date and sign this power of attorney)

I sign my name to this Durable Power of Attorney for Health Care at _____, _____
                                                              (City)   *(State)*

on _____   _____

     (Date)   *(Signature of Principal)*

STATEMENT OF WITNESSES

(This power of attorney will not be valid for making health care decisions unless it is either (1) signed by two qualified adult witnesses who are personally known to you (or to whom you present evidence of your identity) and who are present when you sign or acknowledge your signature or (2) acknowledged before a notary public in California. If you elect to use witnesses rather than a notary public, the law provides that none of the following may be used: (1) the persons you have appointed as your agent and alternate agents, (2) a health care provider or an employee of a health care provider, or (3) an operator or employee of a community care facility or residential care facility for the elderly. Additionally, at least one of the witnesses cannot be related to you by blood, marriage or adoption, or be named in your will. IF YOU ARE A PATIENT IN A SKILLED NURSING FACILITY, ONE OF THE WITNESSES MUST BE A PATIENT ADVOCATE OR OMBUDSMAN.)

I declare under penalty of perjury under the laws of California that the person who signed or acknowledged this document is personally known to me to be the principal, or that the identity of the principal was proved to me by convincing evidence,* that the principal signed or acknowledged this durable power of attorney in my presence, that the principal appears to be of sound mind and under no duress, fraud, or undue influence, that I am not the person appointed as attorney in fact by this document, and that I am not a health care provider, an employee of a health care provider, the operator of a community care facility or a residential care facility for the elderly, nor an employee of an operator of a community care facility or residential care facility for the elderly.

Signature _____

Print name _____

Date _____

Residence Address _____

Signature _____

Print name _____

Date _____

Residence Address _____

(AT LEAST ONE OF THE ABOVE WITNESSES MUST ALSO SIGN THE FOLLOWING DECLARATION)

I further declare under penalty of perjury under the laws of California that I am not related to the principal by blood, marriage, or adoption, and, to the best of my knowledge I am not entitled to any part of the estate of the principal upon the death of the principal under a will now existing or by operation of law.

Signature: _____

---

*The law allows one or more of the following forms of identification as convincing evidence of identity: a California driver's license or identification card or U.S. passport that is current or has been issued within five years, or any of the following if the document is current or has been issued within five years, contains a photograph and description of the person named on it, is signed by the person, and bears a serial or other identifying number: a foreign passport that has been stamped by the U.S. Immigration and Naturalization Service; a driver's license issued by another state or by an authorized Canadian or Mexican agency; or an identification card issued by another state or by any branch of the U.S. armed forces. If the principal is a patient in a skilled nursing facility, a patient advocate or ombudsman may rely on the representations of family members or the administrator or staff of the facility as convincing evidence of identity if the patient advocate or ombudsman believes that the representations provide a reasonable basis for determining the identity of the principal.

SPECIAL REQUIREMENT: STATEMENT OF PATIENT ADVOCATE OR OMBUDSMAN

(If you are a patient in a skilled nursing facility, a patient advocate or ombudsman must sign the Statement of Witnesses above and must also sign the following declaration.)

I further declare under penalty of perjury under the laws of California that I am a patient advocate or ombudsman as designated by the State Department of Aging and am serving as a witness as required by subdivision (f) of Civil Code Section 2432.

Signature: _____   Address: _____

Print Name: _____   _____

Date: _____

CERTIFICATE OF ACKNOWLEDGMENT OF NOTARY PUBLIC

(Acknowledgment before a notary public is not required if you have elected to have two qualified witnesses sign above. If you are a patient in a skilled nursing facility, you must have a patient advocate or ombudsman sign the Statement of Witnesses on page 3 and the Statement of Patient Advocate or Ombudsman above)

State of California   )

)ss.

County of _____)

On this _____ day of _____, in the year _____,

before me, _____,

(here insert name of notary public)

personally appeared _____

(here insert name of principal)

personally known to me (or proved to me on the basis of satisfactory evidence) to be the person whose name is subscribed to this instrument, and acknowledged that he or she executed it. I declare under penalty of perjury that the person whose name is subscribed to this instrument appears to be of sound mind and under no duress, fraud, or undue influence.

NOTARY SEAL

_____

(Signature of Notary Public)

COPIES

YOUR AGENT MAY NEED THIS DOCUMENT IMMEDIATELY IN CASE OF AN EMERGENCY. YOU SHOULD KEEP THE COMPLETED ORIGINAL AND GIVE PHOTOCOPIES OF THE COMPLETED ORIGINAL TO (1) YOUR AGENT AND ALTERNATE AGENTS, (2) YOUR PERSONAL PHYSICIAN, AND (3) MEMBERS OF YOUR FAMILY AND ANY OTHER PERSONS WHO MIGHT BE CALLED IN THE EVENT OF A MEDICAL EMERGENCY. THE LAW PERMITS THAT PHOTOCOPIES OF THE COMPLETED DOCUMENT CAN BE RELIED UPON AS THOUGH THEY WERE ORIGINALS.

Additional forms can be purchased from: Sutter Publications, P.O. Box 7690, San Francisco, CA 94120-7690 • (415) 882-5175

Index

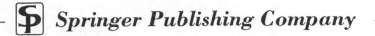 *Springer Publishing Company*

STRATEGIES FOR THERAPY WITH THE ELDERLY
Living with Hope and Meaning

Claire M. Brody, PhD, and **Vicki G. Semel,** PsyD
with a Foreword by **Margot Tallmer,** PhD

This comprehensive volume provides therapy techniques for mental health professionals who work with the elderly. It is also a pragmatic guide for establishing programs and conducting therapy groups in various health settings.

The book covers three major arenas of psychotherapy with the elderly: therapy with people living in nursing homes, with those living in semi-independent housing and participating in community-oriented activities, and with people living independently and seen in private practice. The book's theme is that meaningful therapy can be accomplished with an aging / elderly population in any setting. Stereotypes about aging are confronted with examples of maturation and change through psychotherapy, both individually and in groups.

Contents

I.   **Nursing Homes.** Review of Literature on Working with Staff, Family, and Residents in an Institution. Reminiscence Groups with Women in a Nursing Home. Mothers and Daughters: Caretaking and Adjustment Issues. Working with Residents Who Have Alzheimer's Disease

II. **Community Programs for the Elderly.** Modalities for Working with the Elderly in the Community. Enriched Housing Programs: Developing Strengths in the Frail Elderly. Group Psychotherapy with Depressed Elderly in an Outpatient Treatment Setting

III. **Private Practice.** Individual Treatment of a Rageful, Borderline, Older Woman: The Case of Mrs. Z. Modern Psychoanalytic Therapy with an Aging Male: The Wish for Occupational Success. Private Practice with the Aging Couple: Two Unusual Cases. Countertransference and Ageism: Therapist Reactions to the Older Patient

IV. **Medicare.** A New Political Reality in Treatment: History and Application of Medicare

1993   200pp   0-8261-8010-8   hardcover

536 Broadway, New York, NY 10012-3955 • (212) 431-4370 • Fax (212) 941-7842

SP *Springer Publishing Company*

ENHANCING THE ABILITIES OF PERSONS WITH ALZHEIMER'S AND RELATED DEMENTIAS
A Nursing Perspective

Pam Dawson, RN, MSCN, **Donna Wells,** RN, MHSC, and **Karen Kline,** RN, MScN

The book provides a knowledge foundation for the individualized nursing care of older persons with Alzheimer's disease and related disorders. By way of comprehensive examination of the dementia research literature, the human response to dementia is understood, and specific nursing assessment and caregiving activities are identified and described. The analysis and the interpretation of the research literature is portrayed from an explicit and practical nursing perspective called enablement which focuses attention on the person's abilities or capacities to engage in life as fully as possible despite the unexpected experience of dementia.

Contents:

I. Caring for Persons with Dementia: The Enablement Perspective • What is Enablement? • Enablement and Excess Disability • Enablement and Environmental Press • Enablement and Content for Nursing Practice - Elaboration of the Content Methodology Process

II. Self Care Abilities: Voluntary Movements • Spatial Orientation • Purposeful Movement

III. Social Abilities: Social Cues - Social Contexts

IV. Interactional Abilities: Clinical Features and Threatened Abilities • Comprehension Abilities - Expression Abilities

V. Interpretive Abilities: Recognition - Recall • Subjective Feeling States

1993   184pp   0-8261-7790-5   *hardcover*

536 Broadway, New York, NY 10012-3955 • (212) 431-4370 • Fax (212) 941-7842

Springer Publishing Company

STRESS EFFECTS ON FAMILY CAREGIVERS OF ALZHEIMER'S PATIENTS:
Research and Interventions

Enid Light, PhD,
George Niederehe, PhD,
Barry Lebowitz, PhD, Editors

Facilitates the transfer of research knowledge into clinical practice, service settings and the arena of public policy.

Contents

1994   440pp   08261-7930-4   hardcover

536 Broadway, New York, NY 10012-3955 • (212) 431-4370 • Fax (212) 941-7842